TEAM WORKING & PROFESSIONAL PRACTICE
for Nursing Associates

Sara Miller McCune founded SAGE Publishing in 1965 to support the dissemination of usable knowledge and educate a global community. SAGE publishes more than 1000 journals and over 800 new books each year, spanning a wide range of subject areas. Our growing selection of library products includes archives, data, case studies and video. SAGE remains majority owned by our founder and after her lifetime will become owned by a charitable trust that secures the company's continued independence.

Los Angeles | London | New Delhi | Singapore | Washington DC | Melbourne

SAFINA BIBI
ENRIKA COMLEY
JOANNE FORMAN

TEAM WORKING & PROFESSIONAL PRACTICE

for Nursing Associates

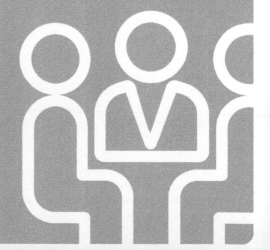

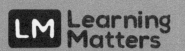

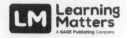

Learning Matters
A SAGE Publishing Company
1 Oliver's Yard
55 City Road
London EC1Y 1SP

SAGE Publications Inc.
2455 Teller Road
Thousand Oaks, California 91320

SAGE Publications India Pvt Ltd
B 1/I 1 Mohan Cooperative Industrial Area
Mathura Road
New Delhi 110 044

SAGE Publications Asia-Pacific Pte Ltd
3 Church Street
#10-04 Samsung Hub
Singapore 049483

Editor: Martha Cunneen
Development editor: Sarah Turpie
Senior project editor: Chris Marke
Project management: River Editorial
Marketing manager: Ruslana Khatagova
Cover design: Wendy Scott
Typeset by: C&M Digitals (P) Ltd, Chennai, India
Printed in the UK

Library of Congress Control Number: 2022945613

British Library Cataloguing in Publication Data

A catalogue record for this book is available from the British Library

ISBN 978-1-5297-6218-1
ISBN 978-1-5297-6217-4 (pbk)

At SAGE we take sustainability seriously. Most of our products are printed in the UK using responsibly sourced papers and boards. When we print overseas we ensure sustainable papers are used as measured by the PREPS grading system. We undertake an annual audit to monitor our sustainability.

Contents

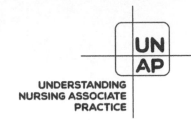

UN
AP

UNDERSTANDING
NURSING ASSOCIATE
PRACTICE

Supporting you through your nursing associate training & career

UNDERSTANDING NURSING ASSOCIATE PRACTICE is a series uniquely designed for trainee nursing associates.

Each book in the series is:

- Mapped to the NMC standards of proficiency for nursing associates
- Affordable
- Full of practical activities & case studies
- Focused on clearly explaining theory & its application to practice

Current books in the series include:

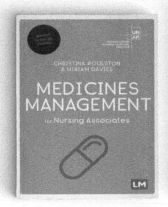

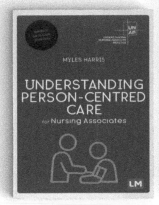

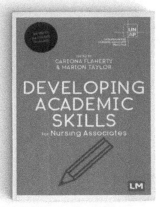

Visit
uk.sagepub.com/UNAP
for more information

About the authors

Safina Bibi is a children's nurse, specialist community public practitioner in school nursing and a registered practice teacher. Currently she is a senior lecturer for the FdSc Nursing Associate Higher Apprenticeship at Birmingham City University (BCU), leading on the Professional Practice module. She had a leading role in the team for quality assurance of the pilot site at BCU for the national development of the nursing associate role. Recently alongside her team she collected the Student Nursing Times Award 2021 for 'Nursing Associate Training Programme Provider of the Year'. Safina is currently studying for her MA in Education, with a keen interest in researching the professional identity of the newly qualified nursing associate in practice.

Enrika Comley is an NMC registered adult nurse and teacher, with a background in general surgery, cardiothoracic surgery and cardiothoracic critical care. She is currently a lecturer at Birmingham City University and has been leading the Leadership/Team Working in Healthcare module for the nursing associates. Enrika has a special interest in human factors and how they contribute to effective team working, and delivering safe care to the service users. Being part of training the first legacy cohort of nursing associates within university has given Enrika an insight into development of the role and the learning needs for the trainees. Enrika is especially passionate about widening participation and supporting learners new to higher education and additional learning needs.

Joanne Forman is a senior lecturer at Birmingham City University and course lead for the FdSc Nursing Associate Higher Apprenticeship. She is a paediatric nurse with a wealth of experience in general paediatrics and surgery and has a specialist degree in Burns and Plastics. She transitioned into Nurse Education working with newly qualified practitioners during preceptorship. She is a Fellow of the Higher Education Academy and is studying for an MA in Education with a specific interest in the widening participation aspects of higher education.

Introduction

Who is this book for?

This book is mainly aimed at trainee nursing associates as it will directly relate to the standards of proficiency that they have to achieve for successful registration and to become an accountable professional. The nursing associate role is a newly regulated profession and this book provides role-specific content that can inform individuals' professional development as they transition into their new profession. It aims to apply to all fields of nursing – adult, children's, mental health and learning disabilities – therefore will be a useful educational reference for a wide range of learners. It may also be of interest to student nurses who would like to develop their understanding of team working and professional practice, especially as nursing associates become part of nursing teams. It may also be useful for lecturers planning their activities and case studies around the subject.

About the book

The nursing associate role will continue to be a new role within healthcare teams for a long time to come, as change requires time. This book will explore how your role fits in within existing healthcare teams and will also introduce you to theories behind the importance of team working. To understand how you will become part of the team, you will first need to reflect on your role and fully understand what it is that you do. There is no single job description, as nursing associates work within different fields of nursing and specialities. We will use reflective activities to help you develop your identity as a nursing associate, which will provide you with confidence in your role, moving forward within your training. NMC *Standards of Proficiency for Nursing Associates* (2018a) are applied throughout the book and specific proficiencies are named within each chapter, relating to the topic. This will help you to understand how each team working and professionalism subject links to your professional practice.

Each chapter has been strategically placed, so that you build on your knowledge as you read it. For example, before you reach Chapter 5, you will be introduced to some ethical and legal frameworks, team working theories and communication methods, where you will be applying this theory to practice. We will focus on developing your knowledge and skills within some of the main skills you will need in practice, some of which will include: prioritisation, delegation, effective communication and raising concerns. You will also be directed to further reading, should you wish to expand your understanding on these topics. This book will promote providing person-centred, safe and compassionate care and the utilisation of evidence-based practice to achieve this. It will also encourage you to consider your own well-being and maintaining your identity, through reflective practice, and continuous professional development.

Book structure

Chapter 1: What is an accountable professional?

This chapter will introduce you to the meaning of professionalism and accountability, relating to the role of the nursing associate. You will explore the difference between a non-professional and professional role, which will help you to understand the transition requirements from your previous role in healthcare, or if this is your first role within the healthcare sector. This chapter will also discuss nursing associate responsibility in duty of candour, actions and omissions, lifelong learning, and maintaining competence and standards of the profession. These terms will then be explored further within the following chapters.

Chapter 2: Understanding what guides your practice

In this chapter, we will focus on demystifying the Nursing Associate Standards of Proficiency, using examples from practice. This chapter will also introduce you to a few essential aspects of becoming a registered professional, including: ethical and legal frameworks as they apply to person-centred care; what is the evidence base and how is this applied to practice; understanding the importance of choice; your own values and beliefs and valuing diversity in practice.

Chapter 3: The interdisciplinary team and how its members influence care

The professional identity and role of the nursing associate within a team will be discussed throughout this chapter. Your role is new to healthcare teams and you may face some challenges at the beginning of your career, but there are many steps that you can take in preparing for becoming part of the team, to smooth the transition. We will therefore discuss the importance of identifying team members and their roles, responsibilities and scope of practice. You will then have an opportunity to complete a few activities relating to communication within teams and how this contributes to the delivery of care. We will also introduce you to an overview of team working theories and how these apply to practice.

Chapter 4: How to deliver and contribute to person-centred care within a team

This chapter is all about understanding how teams collaborate with other healthcare professionals and agencies, while applying principles of person-centred care (PCC). The nursing associate role has been created to enhance the quality of care provided to service users and we will therefore discuss how this can be achieved. This, of course, means that you will be working within a team to identify service user needs, through PCC assessment of their needs and effective communication. We will discuss your role in sharing information with other healthcare professionals, importance of continuous quality improvement activities and advocating for service users.

Chapter 5: Skills for team working

This chapter is all about applying theory to practice. By now we have discussed the theory behind the importance of teamwork and how your role fits within these teams. Here you will be able to dive into case studies to apply your critical thinking skills when it comes to prioritising, delegating, communicating, responding to challenges, understanding professional roles and boundaries, providing constructive feedback to others, contributing to the wider objectives and being a team player; working as a team towards change and sharing the vision, and understanding lines of responsibility.

Chapter 6: How to be heard in difficult situations

Understanding environmental and human factors that influence team working, is an essential part of your role. This chapter will introduce you to the concept of human factors and how they contribute to effective team working, as well as preventing errors occurring. This requires you to develop interpersonal skills to challenge and report errors, near misses, serious incidents and poor practice. It can be very difficult to call out poor practice and report your colleagues, however, it is imperative that you take this responsibility very seriously due to direct, or indirect, impact on service user care. You will therefore develop assertiveness skills to manage working with others and difficult situations through a number of activities and case studies.

Chapter 7: Maintaining your sense of identity and resilience as a nursing associate

Within this chapter, you will examine the importance of self-care and what it means to you as an individual, as well as your professional duty for self-care and seeking support. Recognising stress is an essential skill for a nursing associate to ensure prevention and recognition of 'burnout'. You will therefore be introduced to the concept of emotional intelligence; being aware of and managing your own emotions and the impact of this on service users and your team. You will then identify your own resilience strategy, by exploring a number of examples. Once you have explored your own management of having a healthy lifestyle, we will discuss the importance of acting as a role model and promoting reflection in the development of self and support of others.

Requirements for the NMC: Standards of Proficiency for Nursing Associates

The Nursing and Midwifery Council (NMC) has established standards of proficiency to be met by applicants to different parts of the register, and these are the standards it considers necessary for safe and effective practice. This book is structured so that it will help you to understand and meet the proficiencies required for entry to the NMC register as a nursing associate. The relevant proficiencies are presented at the start of each chapter so that you can clearly see which ones the chapter addresses. The proficiencies have been designed to be generic so they apply to all fields of nursing and all care settings. This is because all nursing associates must be able to meet the needs of any person they encounter in their practice regardless of their stage of life or health challenges, whether these are mental, physical, cognitive or behavioural. Your training to become a nursing associate will be based around meeting these standards through practical and theory assessments. You will then be expected to maintain these standards after you join the NMC register, and revalidate regularly to demonstrate ongoing professional development.

This book includes the latest standards for 2018 onwards, taken from the *Standards of Proficiency for Nursing Associates* (NMC, 2018a).

Learning features

Textbooks can be intimidating and learning from reading text is not always easy. However, this series has been designed specifically to help the nursing associate learn from the books within it. By using a number of learning features throughout the books, they will help you to develop your understanding and ability to apply theory to practice, while remaining engaging and breaking the text up into manageable chunks. This book contains activities, case studies, theory summary boxes, further reading, useful websites and other materials to enable you to participate in your own learning. The book cannot provide all the answers – but instead provides a good outline of the most important information and helps you build a framework for your own learning.

While it would be useful to read this book from beginning to end, you can also access relevant chapters only throughout your training. You may find that you come back to different chapters as your knowledge and practice develops, so that you can access further reading and reflect on your new skills. Team working and professional practice are subjects requiring continuous reflection and improvement, as you will often change teams you are working with or change your speciality. You will be able to come back to further reading lists and references, as you advance within your training.

You will probably find that learning from case studies and scenarios will be most beneficial to you, helping you to develop critical thinking skills, which then can be applied in your everyday practice. Scenarios within this book have been chosen to address everyday challenges that nursing associates have been facing within their roles. This will prepare you for possible situations you might find yourself in and equip you with skills for effective communication with your team.

Final word

Starting a new career can be very daunting and most likely overwhelming. It is okay to have these feelings and it is okay to take your time in developing your skills and knowledge. Everyone within the teams that you will work with will also be developing and learning something, as there is always something new to learn within healthcare! This means that you are all in the same boat and must support one another. Supporting colleagues is a big part of NMC standards and everyone has a responsibility to ensure they are an effective team member. Most importantly, this is essential for the safe and effective person-centred care that we provide. We hope that you will find the information and tips in this book useful to support your academic studies, practice and to aid your development as a nursing associate. We also hope that all the books within this series will help you to develop confidence, patience and self-awareness within your practice. We wish you all the best with your studies!

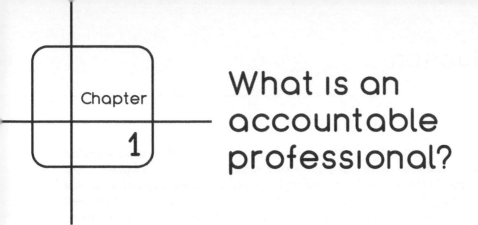

Chapter 1

What is an accountable professional?

NMC STANDARDS OF PROFICIENCY FOR NURSING ASSOCIATES

This chapter will address the following platforms and proficiencies:

Platform 1: Being an accountable professional

At the point of registration, the registered nursing associate will be able to:

1.1   understand and act in accordance with The Code: Professional Standards of Practice and Behaviour for Nurses, Midwives and Nursing Associates, and fulfil all registration requirements

1.2   understand and apply relevant legal, regulatory and governance requirements, policies, and ethical frameworks, including any mandatory reporting duties, to all areas of practice

1.3   understand the importance of courage and transparency and apply the duty of candour, recognising and reporting any situations, behaviours or errors that could result in poor care outcomes

1.16   act as an ambassador for their profession and promote public confidence in health and care services

Chapter aims

After reading this chapter, you will be able to:

- understand what it means to be an accountable professional;
- identify the parameters of practice for the nursing associate;
- understand the differences between a regulated and non-regulated profession;
- explain how competence can be maintained.

Introduction

Case study: Stephanie

A nurse who had been qualified for eight years had to account for her actions at a disciplinary hearing to the NMC after she gave a dialysis patient a sugary drink instead of a glucose drip. During the inquest she also admitted to committing a series of errors including not knowing the difference between milligrams and micrograms and checking a patient's temperature instead of blood pressure. Other allegations included numerous drug administration errors including giving medications to patients when she was not authorised to do so, preparing drugs for a nil-by-mouth patient and attempting to give drugs that had already been given. The NMC Conduct and Competence Committee also heard that the nurse was unfamiliar with equipment on a resuscitation trolley.

Her fitness to practise was found to be impaired by reason of lack of competence. She was given a 12-month suspension order.

Activity 1.1   Reflection

Write down the issues raised in the above case study.

Have you ever been put in a position where you have felt that you were working outside your level of competence?

As this answer is based on your own reflection, no outline answer is provided at the end of this chapter.

As a registered nursing associate, the need for maintaining competence and standards of the profession means that you will be accountable for all actions you undertake and those where you fail to do so. This chapter begins by exploring areas such as professional practice and the underpinning principles of this. You will be guided through defining terms such as 'professionalism' and 'accountability' and relating this to the role of the nursing associate. The difference between a non-professional and professional role will provide you with a basis to understand the transition and changing expectations from a non-regulated role to a regulated role within healthcare. The chapter will conclude with a discussion around duty of candour.

The Code (NMC, 2018b) requires students to demonstrate professional values, ability to communicate effectively, contribute to integrated care while putting the best interests and preferences of those they care for first. Such practice can only be achieved if the fundamental concept of 'professionalism' is clearly understood as good health outcomes are highly dependent on the professional practice and behaviours of the individual delivering it.

Professionalism in practice

Professionalism can mean many things to many people, but it is better understood once you have an understanding of the term profession. Profession has been defined as a chosen, paid, occupation that requires training and formal qualification (Behrend et al., 2006). Therefore, professionals are individuals who are expected to demonstrate skills and behaviours in accordance with their profession. For nursing associates, defining the term requires an understanding of two key fundamental professional standards that govern the practice of the nursing associate. Like registered nurses, who are governed by *The Code* (NMC, 2018b), nursing associates have additional standards published by the NMC, which set out the knowledge, competencies, professional behaviours and behaviours expected of them when they join the register. The *Standards of Proficiencies for Nursing Associates* (NMC, 2018a) alongside *The Code* (NMC, 2018b) emphasise the need to promote professionalism and trust through the values set out in both standards. Acting with honesty and integrity not only allows the practice of recognising and reporting behaviours that could result in poor care outcomes, but leads to confidence and trust in the profession from those it intends to protect. Essentially, upholding individual professionalism and the reputation of the profession, all registered nursing associates are required to practise within their limits of competence utilising evidence-based practice to inform their practice.

To gain a further understanding of *The Code* in relation to competence, it is imperative to recognise that you are to uphold *The Code* within the limits of your competence. This means, while working alongside a nurse delivering an aspect of care, you will uphold the standards in *The Code* within the contribution you make to overall care. The professional commitment to work within one's competence is a key underlying principle of the professional standard. If the above fundamental characteristics are not upheld and fall below expected professional requirements, nursing associates will be held accountable for their actions. Accountability is fundamentally linked to the concept of professionalism, where you are answerable for your actions or omissions to a regulating body. This will be further explored later in the chapter.

Principles of professional practice

The purpose of professionalism for nursing associates is essentially to ensure consistent provision of safe, effective care for people of all ages across the four fields of nursing, namely, working with adults, children, learning disability and mental health patients. Let's now examine aspects of behaviour, attitude and approaches that underpin good care.

Integrity

Case study: Sam

Sam, a trainee nursing associate, is on placement at an adult surgical ward caring for an elderly patient post-operation. It is very busy on the ward and she is also supporting her practice assessor with other patients. With her allocated elderly patient she has been delegated to monitor the patient's vital signs and assist with his activities of daily living. At the end of the shift Sam realises that she should have assessed the patient's vital signs every four hours, but they were only assessed once that shift. Since the patient is now resting quietly, and seems stable, Sam falsifies the data and enters fabricated vital signs to comply with the every-four-hour assessment. At handover, to her practice assessor, Sam states the vital signs were stable. When the practice assessor asks if she assessed them every four hours, she states that she did.

From the above case study, the trainee fails to demonstrate honesty in the patient relationship by documenting false information, and by failing to communicate honest information with the practice assessor. There will be times in practice that you are working under constant pressure in fast-paced environments with understaffed resources, however, a commitment to understanding integrity is paramount. In the above case study, the implication of falsifying the patient's vital signs means not only is the patient at risk of clinical deterioration but it also questions the lack of integrity in Sam's behaviour. Integrity can be viewed as behaviours which include providing honest information to the patient and public, honest and accurate documentation of patient care, reporting errors made by self and others and most importantly, demonstrating the ability to uphold these at all times.

Activity 1.2   Critical thinking

Before reading further, make a list of behaviours that you think are devoid of integrity. Remember to include behaviours that an individual may display in the academic setting too.

As this answer is based on your own observation, no outline answer is provided at the end of this chapter.

Having considered behaviours that are devoid of integrity, you may have included the following in your critical thinking: cheating, plagiarism, lying and deception. Integrity as a behaviour for the trainee nursing associate encompasses honesty not only in clinical practice but in the academic setting as well.

Academic integrity

Academic integrity has been described as professional conduct that demonstrates ethical behaviour in the education setting (Devine and Chin, 2018). This professional conduct alludes to ethical behaviours set out in the professional standards that clearly require the trainee nursing associate to engage in honest behaviour even at the backdrop of the demands of professional practice. As a work-based learner, the demands of learning in 'two worlds' – that of the university and clinical practice – means the experience is very different to traditional nursing programmes. While there is a physical distinction between the two settings, the behaviours you demonstrate in clinical practice should be a continuum of the behaviours demonstrated in the academic setting.

Case study: Ahmed

Ahmed is a trainee nursing associate in his second year of training. He has been struggling with time management recently with assignment deadlines, looking after his ill mother and attending work. He has an assignment deadline approaching and he is worried that he will not be able to complete the assignment in time for submission. He has worked extremely hard academically and feels that for his next submission, approaching a fellow colleague who is a registered nursing associate, will provide him with the support he needs. He asks the nursing associate to share the assignment she submitted for guidance. Ahmed intentionally copies parts of the assignment and submits this as his own work. Ahmed feels this is only a one-off as he has been under stress with the demanding workload in the clinical environment.

The above case study illustrates many factors that may have played in Ahmed ultimately making the decision to cheat and plagiarise. Ahmed may have justified his actions relating to:

Internal factors:

- *Individual character* and what he feels is acceptable or unacceptable behaviour. This is closely related to professional ethics which will be discussed in a later chapter. However, for Ahmed, he has accepted it is acceptable to cheat. He is morally aware of the decision between right and wrong.
- *Accountability* or lack of accountability and taking ownership of the action itself. Ahmed has accounted the reason for copying as a result of his demanding workload, thus not taking any responsibility for the action.

External factors:

- *Organisational influences* such as the sheer volume of work in the clinical practice has contributed to feelings of stress and being overworked.
- *Support systems* have been recognised in the case study as his colleague provides him with her previous work. However, the expectations of this support have been misused by Ahmed.
- *Academic workload* and the inability to effectively manage the balance of academic life along with the expectations of working and complexities of family life.

The concern is if Ahmed continues to believe this act of cheating is somehow justified, then this behaviour may certainly continue in his professional practice once he is a qualified professional.

Activity 1.3   Reflection

Which individuals and/or organisations do you think Ahmed's behaviour has a direct impact on?
As this answer is based on your own reflection, no outline answer is provided at the end of this chapter.

Now that you have reflected on the above, were you able to identify the following affected stakeholders?

- *Academic institution:* plagiarising in any form could be considered a breach of *The Code* as in this case, Ahmed has acted dishonestly. He risks an investigation for academic misconduct at an institutional level with possible long-term implications for his misconduct once he has completed his studies.
- *Employer:* Ahmed is a work-based learner who is contractually employed which means he is directly accountable to his employer for his behaviour with possible disciplinary or cautionary sanctions put in place.
- *Registered nursing associate:* the person that gave Ahmed her work for support is a victim of theft as her words were taken without consent.

- *Patient/public:* dishonesty in professional practice places the public and patient at risk. Provision of quality and safe patient care depends on a foundation of honest attainment of academic achievement.

This discussion should have provided you with an insight into the importance of demonstrating and maintaining integrity as a trainee nursing associate in the classroom and clinical environment and the possible consequences if this behaviour is not adhered to. In order to qualify as a registered nursing associate, there is a requirement from the academic institution you have studied with to provide a statement of good character at the end of the programme. *The Code* clearly states the requirement of upholding the reputation of the profession. Any behaviours that contradict the reputation of the profession will consequently impact on your ability to be registered by the Nursing and Midwifery Council.

Fitness to practise

The Nursing and Midwifery Council regulate the role of the nursing associate. This means the regulator has a legal responsibility to ensure protection of the public from substandard care by the healthcare professionals its organisation registers. Fitness to practise is the ability to meet the profession's standards as set by the regulator. It is your responsibility to ensure that you understand why the professional standards are important and your role in achieving fitness to practise. The role the NMC plays in achieving fitness to practise is to safeguard the public's confidence in the nursing and midwifery profession by promoting the health, safety and well-being of the public through maintaining the professional standards.

Examples of issues that may lead to fitness to practise proceedings:

- misconduct;
- lack of competence;
- criminal behaviour;
- serious ill health;
- determinations by other health and social care organisations.

There is a misconception that fitness to practise proceedings are there as a punitive measure. It is important to understand the key role of the NMC is to protect the public. Therefore, such investigations are about managing risks that the nursing associate poses to patients or members of the public in the future. It is not about punishing individuals for past events. What do you think is the risk if nursing associates see fitness to practise proceedings as a punitive measure? When answering this question you may have thought about the risk of professionals not being open and honest when things do go wrong. The risk of being punished may deter individuals from being transparent. Nursing associates who admit to mistakes being made need to be encouraged to engage with their professional duty of candour which promotes an open culture of learning. We know deliberately covering up when things go wrong seriously undermines patient safety and damages public trust in the profession.

Fitness to practise referrals are triggered by complaints and allegations referred to the NMC: these referrals can come from patients, colleagues, police, employers and other regulators. It is not uncommon for individuals to 'self-refer'; this will usually happen when individuals notify the NMC about convictions and cautions.

Activity 1.4   Critical thinking

Access the NMC guidance on fitness to practise outcomes by accessing the link https://www.nmc.org.uk/concerns-nurses-midwives/what-is-fitness-to-practise/fitness-to-practise-outcomes/
Read the overview of the possible outcomes following a fitness to practise hearing. Now make a list of the five possible sanctions. On further exploration you will find not all proceedings may progress to a full hearing. When do you think this happens?

An outline answer is provided at the end of the chapter.

The sanctions discussed are based on a series of factors that determine the seriousness of the outcomes placed. As a nursing associate it is important to have awareness of the reasons why individuals may be referred. One of the issues that may lead to a referral is lack of competence, which is explored further below.

Competency and standards of the profession

While the *Standards of Proficiency for Nursing Associates* (NMC, 2018a) provide clarity around the role to diminish any blurring of professional boundaries and responsibilities, the importance of ensuring competence and proficiency before undertaking any task, no matter how experienced you are, is fundamental. Competency is a key principle of *The Code*, and without it patient safety is at risk. The uniqueness of the role means those training to become registered nursing associates may have been previously employed in healthcare in a different unregulated role for varying years. The scope of practice for unregulated roles differs between organisations which means there are no standards for education for these roles. These essential supporting roles (healthcare assistants, support workers, link workers to name a few) will undertake competency-based skills training to practise in their respective role. For you as a nursing associate it is imperative to understand and recognise the increased accountability for a regulated profession when practising. Takase and Teraoka (2011) define competency as a set of attributes that fulfil an individual's responsibility through practice. These attributes are personal characteristics, professional attitude, values, knowledge and skills. As a nursing associate, the ability (competence) to develop competency, which is the behavioural action you undertake, you need to have the mentioned attributes present. Let's look at this closer in relation to your specific standards. The *Standards of Proficiency for Nursing Associates* (NMC, 2018a) set out the knowledge, skills and attributes that all nursing associates must demonstrate when caring for people of all ages and across all health and care settings. In order to achieve this, education institutions provide an education programme that meet these standards. Without the learning that is provided by the education institution attended, nursing associates will not be able to gain the ability to develop competency to perform their duties competently. The following case study activity will give you the opportunity to identify the attributes that make the competent practitioner.

Case study: Marion

Marion is in Year 1 of her nursing associate apprenticeship, she has been at her current placement at the GP surgery for four weeks. This is Marion's first placement working with adults. Shaid, a 40-year-old man, has attended the surgery to have his sutures removed following surgery ten days ago. The registered nurse who is going to remove the sutures leaves the room to get missing equipment, while Marion is asked to remove the wound dressing by the registered nurse. Marion asks Shaid how he thinks his wound has been healing. Shaid shares with Marion that he has been extremely anxious following his surgery and wants more information about the impact of his surgical procedure. He has had some support at home to change his dressing but has been in pain most of the time. During this point, Marion is removing the dressing and recognises unhealthy granulation at the base of the wound. Shaid asks Marion about the wound. This is the first time following her skills session at university she has observed a wound. She is unsure if the wound is healing or if there is a presence of infection. She tells Shaid the nurse will be here who can assess the wound alongside her and will be able to give him more information. Marion does ponder for a moment whether to tell Shaid about the unhealthy granulation, but she recognises that it would be unprofessional to give Shaid the wrong information before a clinical discussion had taken place with the nurse. She actively listens to Shaid while he shares his feelings of anxiety and reassures him that she will access his medical notes when the nurse has removed the sutures to go through the information he has requested. Once the nurse returns, Marion explains her assessment of the wound and why she thinks there might be a possible infection.

Activity 1.5   Reflection and critical thinking

Which personal characteristics did Marion display when she was engaging with Shaid?
 Do you think Marion demonstrated a professional attitude by not sharing a suspected possible infection at the wound bed?
 How did Marion demonstrate competence?
 An outline answer is provided at the end of the chapter.

Providing care based on professional knowledge and skills includes being able to collaborate with other healthcare professionals to support clinical decision making. Therefore, competency can be seen as a complex integration of knowledge, skills and values including professional judgement which Marion displays. In the case study Marion's competence is influenced by the theoretical underpinning knowledge she has obtained from the higher education institute where she was provided with the theory around wound assessment. She then applies this theory in practice to develop her competency. However, it is important to recognise competence is not constant: this means it can change and develop over time.

Maintaining competence

To fulfil registration requirements once qualified as a nursing associate, it is an expectation that all nursing associates must keep their knowledge up to date, taking part in regular learning and professional development activities to develop competence. Maintaining competence is a continuous process; it does not end once you have gained a professional qualification. Healthcare practices are underpinned by evidence-based practice. This means as a practitioner you will be expected to continually re-evaluate your competence so clinical decisions made are based on best available, current, valid and relevant evidence. So how can you maintain competence?

Additional support: Your role as a nursing associate is working in four fields of nursing across specialities, therefore you will need to ask for extra support or complete additional competency training to work with confidence in the area of practice that you are not familiar with.

Continuing professional development (CPD): This is a requisite to maintaining competence: not only does it enhance personal skills such as boosting confidence, but it is an investment you make in yourself. It also allows enhancement of professionalism by improving the quality of nursing care you will provide. The ability to devote time to continuing professional development can at times be challenging but negotiating learning time with employers is recommended. CPD in the public sector (NHS) is usually paid by the employer with in-house training. For those who work in the independent sector (non-NHS) regulations are less well-established in regard to CPD. Consequently, there is a risk CPD may not be given as much priority compared to the public sector. Regardless of this, the NMC requires that all registrants (both public and independent) meet its CPD requirements through revalidation.

What type of activities count towards CPD?

- Attending conferences, webinars, online learning modules and meetings – networking with other healthcare professionals, learning from researchers.
- Structured professional clinical supervision – this can develop your critical thinking and problem-solving skills.
- Reading and reviewing publications – this supports an awareness of clinical practice developments and how they can impact on the care you provide to patients.

The above is not an exhaustive list but provides you with some understanding of some of the activities that can form part of the revalidation process to maintain and develop competence.

What does accountability mean?

To start thinking about the meaning of accountability, let's have a look at the below case study.

Case study: Responsibility vs. accountability

Rosie is a healthcare assistant who has recently joined a busy surgical ward in an acute hospital. She has had no previous healthcare experience, however, she has now completed a hospital induction training for the role. She is working on a shift with Adam, who has been a registered nursing associate for three months now. At the start of the shift, Adam asks Rosie if she wouldn't mind preparing Michael's (patient) for heart surgery, by ensuring that his chest and legs are shaved (this aims to minimise risk of infection during and after the operation). Rosie nods and starts her day on the ward. However, as the morning progresses, Rosie feels overwhelmed with many different tasks on the ward and forgets to shave Michael's chest and legs. Theatre staff arrive to collect the patient and it becomes clear that the patient was not prepared for surgery, thus delaying the start of the surgery and all subsequent procedures for that day. Although the

(Continued)

(Continued)

patient does not mind and understands how busy the ward staff were, the theatre charge nurse complains about Adam to his manager.

Adam ensures that his patient is then prepared for surgery as soon as possible and attends the manager's office, to discuss what has happened.

The above case study is a perfect example of accountability and responsibility of those caring for service users. Although in this case, no harm was caused to the patient, it is fair to say that if a more important task was missed, it could have serious consequences for the patient.

Activity 1.6   Discussion

Consider Rosie and Adam's case study above. Who do you think was responsible for this error occurring? Why do you think it is Adam who has been called to the manager's office and not Rosie?

Complete this activity to develop your understanding between accountability and responsibility.

An outline answer is provided at the end of this chapter.

You may be used to taking responsibility in everyday life. This can come in many different shapes and forms, such as paying bills on time or putting the rubbish bin outside ready for the collection day. These tasks are still called responsibilities, however, the consequences of making an error in these situations are not usually catastrophic, and changes can be made to resolve it by accepting the late payment fee or taking rubbish to the local tip. In healthcare, this becomes more complicated and if a mistake is made, such as in the above case study, someone is held responsible for the error, having to accept the consequences for it.

Definition of responsibility is

a duty to deal with or take care of somebody/something, so that you may be blamed if something goes wrong (Oxford Dictionary, 2020).

In the above scenario, Rosie was responsible for completing the task allocated and could be simply blamed for this, however Adam was ultimately accountable for delegating this task, due to being a registered practitioner. Delegation is a big part of the nursing associate's role, especially when working within interdisciplinary teams. We will be covering teamwork later in this book, where we will explore concepts of delegation in more detail.

Platform 1 of the NMC *Standards of Proficiency for Nursing Associates* (2018a) states that nursing associates must always act professionally, while using their knowledge, skills and attitudes to make evidence-based decisions. These decisions must be made in the best interest of the people, in collaboration with them, while recognising the parameters of their role.

This means that Adam was required to understand the risks and benefits of delegating this task, while using his experience to ensure he follows up the completion of the task delegated, especially to a colleague who was new in their role. It is important to highlight that Adam was not accountable for the delegatee's actions, however he did not overlook the completion of the task, and this he was accountable for. The NMC *Code* (2018b) helps nursing associates to take correct steps when delegating tasks, by highlighting the importance of assessing the most competent person to complete the task, thus taking professional responsibility overall.

Avoiding the blame culture

When considering the above definition of responsibility, it would be easy to conclude that it is always the healthcare professional's 'fault' if something goes wrong somewhere along the service user's care journey. However, this would be a very narrow view approach, leading to minimal learning and development. Understanding accountability means that healthcare professionals have the required skills to consider all arguments for and against, before making a decision, thus reducing the risk of the decision being harmful. Taking away the opportunity to learn from the mistakes means that instead of ensuring this does not happen again, healthcare professionals take on full consequences and the blame. It is also important to consider other factors, which contribute to errors occurring, besides the capabilities of the healthcare professional. To ensure continuous learning, a safety culture must be established, where healthcare professionals and the organisation are open to investigating the root cause of errors, which may not lead to one individual's 'fault' (Chaffer, 2016). These are human factors principles, which help us to understand the interaction between the professional and the problem they are presented with. We will be covering the concept of human factors later in the book, where we discuss the importance of patient safety and avoiding errors in practice.

Activity 1.7 Reflection

Consider a time when you had to take accountability for your actions. This can be a situation from your everyday life or a healthcare setting. Pay particular attention to why you chose to own up to your mistakes and take responsibility and the consequences. What standards or values influenced this?

An outline answer is provided at the end of this chapter.

Why is accountability important to you?

Being an accountable professional means that service users are able to put their trust in you and always expect their care needs to be handled based on high standards of evidence-based knowledge and skills. They should also be able to expect that nursing associates are following clear guidelines, law and legislation, to always provide a high standard of care. This expectation also extends to the trainee nursing associates, who should be aware of their responsibility in upholding professional standards. However, accountability is not only important for the service users; nursing associates must be supported by regulatory bodies, such as the NMC, who provide guidance to ensure strict parameters of limitations to professional roles. This means that you, as a nursing associate, have a clear understanding of what your responsibilities are in upholding standards of proficiency for being an accountable professional. Baillie and Black (2014) suggests that by maintaining transparency in your decision making about actions and outcomes of care delivery, you are demonstrating your accountability. Having confidence to provide a rationale (explanation) for your actions will therefore not only help you make better decisions in practice but also ensure patient safety.

One of the most common issues faced by the trainee nursing associates and registered nursing associates is still the perception of the role and its remit. To understand the impact of Introduction of Nursing Associates, Health Education England (HEE) conducted an evaluation report, which was split into Phase 1 and Phase 2 (2018). HEE reported on the factors that helped or hindered progression of the role. Amongst the factors associated with academic ability and establishing a successful home-work-study balance, one of the main issues remained in existing healthcare professionals understanding the role of NA, and their responsibilities. For the TNAs and NAs this continues to cause problems in integrating within nursing teams, due to lack of understanding and trust, a key reported problem being in understanding the differences between NA and RN roles.

Table 1.1 outlines the main similarities and differences between the two roles. While some of the roles, such as being an accountable professional, health promotion and patient safety, are the same, there are clear differences in delivery of care. The table highlights that NAs will be contributing to key aspects of service user care, however the RNs will be co-ordinating this care and taking the lead in ensuring all aspects of complex care delivery are managed appropriately. It is important to remember that this will look different, depending on which healthcare setting the NA is working within and number of additional competencies completed. On completion of registered nurse training, nurses will be trained in one of the four fields of nursing, compared to NAs, who are generic practitioners, with understanding of all four fields of nursing and how they influence the delivery of person-centred care. Understanding the differences between the two roles will aid your development in becoming an accountable professional, aware of the parameters of your role.

Table 1.1 Main role differences between nursing associates and registered nurses (Adapted from: Nursing and Midwifery Council, 2019)

Nursing associate 6 platforms	Registered nurse 7 platforms
Be an accountable professional	Be an accountable professional
Promoting health and preventing ill health	Promoting health and preventing ill health
Provide and monitor care	**Provide and evaluate care**
(NA's are required to have essential knowledge and skills to monitor service user care and recognise any concerns, which may need escalating)	(RN's must not only recognise deterioration and monitor progress, but also determine the significance of any changes observed)
Working in teams	**Leading and managing nursing care and working in teams**
(NA's are required to work within multidisciplinary teams and may take lead within specific tasks, however, will not be leading and managing overall team goals)	(RN's are required to take lead in planning teams' approach to nursing care delivery)
Improving safety and quality of care	Improving safety and quality of care
Contributing to integrated care	**Coordinating care**
(Looking at the example across, NA may be part of the team in organising complex care needs for the service user, may conduct some of the referrals, where appropriate, however would not be taking charge or overlooking the whole complex discharge. The weighing of the contribution to integrated care may change, depending on the competence level of additional training)	(RN's may be required to ensure that care is delivered seamlessly between different healthcare services. For example, overlooking the discharge of a service user into the community setting with complex needs. This could involve multiple referrals and coordination of appointments, to ensure interdisciplinary approach)
	Assessing needs and planning care
	(On completion of RN training, they are equipped with skills and knowledge to assess service user care needs and recognise key aspects of planning to provide excellent quality of care)

What is duty of candour?

So far, we have discussed what it means to be a professional, especially as the role of the nursing associate has become regulated by the NMC. We also explored the meaning behind accountability, which is often mistaken for responsibility. Being accountable for all your actions can feel overwhelming at times, as we fear making the wrong decision, which could lead to a mistake and it may, or may not harm the patient. But errors in practice are inevitable and sometimes do affect patient outcomes. These can be short- or long-term effects and unfortunately, can even lead to death.

Part of being a registered and accountable professional is informing the service user (or/and Next of Kin (NOK)) of the error that has occurred. To understand this further, let's have a look at the example below.

Case study: Remi

Remi is a TNA, working alongside Dom (registered NA) in a specialist dementia nursing home. Remi has previously worked within a mental health setting and only recently started his new role within the adult nursing field. This meant that Remi was used to the service users being mostly mobile and independent with their activities of daily living. This was not the case at the dementia nursing home, where the majority of the residents required physical care, such as for hygiene, mobilisation and skincare. This was a learning curve for Remi and he worked under the close supervision of Dom, to ensure that he completed required tasks appropriately and documented care accurately.

However, after a busy few shifts in the week, Remi was approached by his practice assessor Dom, to have a conversation about one of the residents who they had looked after during the week. Unfortunately, it appeared that the patient had developed a grade 2 pressure ulcer and it appeared to have happened during the last couple of shifts, when Dom was in charge of the resident's care. Remi knew that he was responsible for updating the skin/rotation documentation over the last couple of shifts and was worried that he had made a mistake, although he thought that he was up to date with it and had also provided the required care. He was still unsure though, as he was still new to the role and feared that his lack of knowledge could have led to the skin damage.

Dom explained to Remi that although it appeared that all required care was provided to the resident, they had still developed a pressure ulcer while in their care. Further investigation will take place to determine if the pressure ulcer development could have been prevented or not. However, while the investigation occurs, Dom now has a duty of candour to inform the resident and their NOK what has happened and apologise for any potential consequence/treatment required.

Activity 1.8   Reflection and critical thinking

Remi has not experienced a situation like this before and plans to research the concept of 'duty of candour' in more detail, and to write a reflective account, evaluating his actions and learning in this situation.

Consider the following questions, based on the case study above:

(Continued)

(Continued)

1. Who do you think was accountable for the resident acquiring a pressure sore?
2. If you were in Remi's situation, would you feel like it was your fault? Why? Why not?
3. Do you think Dom is right in saying that they must apologise to the patient (and/or NOK)?
4. Does this mean they are taking legal responsibility for what has happened?

An outline answer is provided at the end of this chapter.

It is paramount that we continue trying to prevent errors from happening in practice, which hopefully means less harm caused to patients. When errors do occur, healthcare professionals must remain accountable for their actions. In the above case study, Dom (registered NA) is accountable for the care provided to the patient, while looking after them during the period they acquired a pressure sore. There are many reasons why a patient may develop a pressure ulcer, including lack of mobility, cognitive impairment, malnutrition and lack of hydration amongst some of the examples (NICE, 2015). However, as it was acquired while in care, we must take responsibility by being open and honest with the patient.

Duty of candour means that the healthcare professional needs to be open and honest with patients (or/and NOK) when something goes wrong, leading to harm or potential harm (NMC, 2015). This is part of NA professional responsibility and must be upheld as soon as possible, after the incident has occurred. There are three steps that we must take when complying with duty of candour (see Figure 1.1): these steps should then be followed by an apology.

1. Tell the patient (or/and NOK) when something has gone wrong. This should be done as soon as possible.	2. If possible, offer an appropriate solution and provide support required.	3. Explain to the patient (or/and NOK) the details of has happened and potential consequences/next steps.

Figure 1.1 Steps to meet responsibility for duty of candour

Apologising does not mean that the individual is legally liable for what has happened. Receiving an apology for what has happened is essential for high-quality person-centred care and should not be mistaken for taking personal legal responsibility, which could be held against them in court. Therefore, if you have made an error that has affected the patient, it is always best to first seek support from your senior management colleagues but also you should not be afraid to apologise. NMC (2015) do highlight that an apology does not necessarily need to always come from the individual who has caused harm/potential harm, but a face-to-face apology from someone within the organisation is usually appreciated and helps towards resolving the situation.

You can learn more about duty of candour by accessing joint guidance from the NMC and General Medical Council (GMC) by following the link at the end of this chapter. It provides you with further rationale on why duty of candour is important and details on the steps you will need to take.

Chapter summary

This chapter provides you with an overview of what it means to be an accountable professional as a nursing associate. You have been guided through the importance of the professional standards and how these guide your practice. If you are unsure what you are permitted to do, discuss this with your practice supervisors or line manager. The key differences between a registered nurse and a registered nursing associate have been explored: this knowledge will now give you the opportunity to understand the key role of your profession in healthcare. You will be able to work across the four fields of nursing, therefore it is your responsibility to familiarise yourself and adhere to the local policy of the organisation that you are working for. In doing so, you will be demonstrating the key knowledge, skills and behaviours that you need to practise as a safe nursing associate. The activity tools used in this chapter are a starting point in getting you to reflect and critically think about your professional standards when applied in the practice setting, but always remember developing knowledge is a continuous skill that will continue in your workplace.

Activities: Brief outline answers

Activity 1.4 Critical thinking (page 11)

The five possible sanctions include:

1. No sanction
2. Caution order
3. Conditions of practice order
4. Suspension order
5. Striking-off order

Other ways that cases can end include resolving cases by agreement. If a nursing associate wants to resolve their case by agreement, they must accept the facts outlined in the concern and accept that their fitness to practise is impaired. This is undertaken under a consensual panel determination, whereby an appropriate sanction is agreed upon. A nursing associate can also apply for voluntary removal from the register if they are being investigated before going to a full investigation.

Activity 1.5 Reflection and critical thinking (page 12)

Which personal characteristics did Marion display when she was engaging with Shaid?

Marion was understanding when Shaid discussed his anxieties; she listened to him and was also able to problem solve by offering a solution to reducing his anxieties in answering the questions when his medical records were accessed. She also exercised self-control. While Marion had undertaken a skills and knowledge session at university in wound assessment, this was her first wound observation therefore she adhered to Annex A of the *Standards of Proficiencies for Nursing Associates* where skill 2.7 states *address and respond to people's questions, recognising when to refer to others in order to provide accurate response.*

Do you think Marion demonstrated a professional attitude by not sharing that she suspected a possible infection at the wound bed?

Marion demonstrated being aware of her own limitations. While she had been delegated to take the dressing off, she uses her knowledge about wound assessment and assesses the possibility of the wound being infected. However, she also recognises while she has the knowledge, she has not undertaken the competency of wound assessment and takes the professional responsibility of collaborating with the registered nurse to make this assessment.

How did Marion demonstrate competence?

Marion demonstrated competence by understanding what was being asked of her when she was delegated the task of taking off the dressing and preparing for the sutures to be removed. She can provide a rationale to the nurse as to why she has assessed the wound to be possibly infected. She has identified unhealthy granulation and can provide knowledge in regard to this but does not share this information with Shaid because it is the first time she has assessed a wound and needs support to undertake a full assessment. She uses the skill of effective communication to listen to Shaid and is honest when he asks questions about the wound.

Activity 1.6 Discussion (page 14)

One possible answer for this discussion point is that both Rosie and Adam were responsible for not ensuring that patient X had been fully prepared for surgery. Both Rosie and Adam should reflect on their actions and responsibilities as healthcare employers. However, Adam is called to the manager's office because he was the registered nursing associate delegating the task to his colleague. Adam has accountability towards this task and will now need to discuss the consequences of this going wrong with the manager. This type of error usually means having to reflect on the actions taken, looking at the professional responsibilities of safe delegation and making an action plan to avoid this happening in the future.

Activity 1.7 Reflection (page 15)

There is no right or wrong situation to reflect on, as reflection is a personal technique to evaluate your own actions and other factors that impacted on that situation. You may consider a time when you took responsibility for your actions, due to feeling guilty about how your actions affected others. Your personal values and employer values may have impacted on your decision to admit your error and take responsibility. It is important to consider what you have learned from the situation and how this will influence your future decisions.

Activity 1.8 Reflection and critical thinking (page 17)

1. Hopefully you have considered that Dom would be the NA accountable for what has happened, as the pressure ulcer was acquired while the patient was in his care. There may be other individuals involved in what has happened, or no one at all as the resident may have acquired the pressure ulcer due to other factors besides someone making an error. However, Dom had to be able to discuss the documentation completed throughout the shifts and at which point the pressure ulcer developed, which was not very clear. While Remi was asked to complete the documentation, Dom needed to closely supervise Remi and ensure that correct actions were taken.

2. You may have answered that you would feel like it was your fault, as you did not feel confident in completing the documentation or still felt anxious being new to the area of practice. It is important to highlight that you should never complete any tasks that you do not feel confident and competent in doing. This is part of your professional standards and recognising your own limitations to practise helps to maintain patient safety.

3. As discussed earlier in the chapter, apologising to the patient (or/and NOK) does not mean that individual is taking personal legal responsibility for what has happened, but rather providing person-centred care and apologising that the incident has happened which has caused harm/potential harm and possibly affected their outcome or length of treatment. It shows compassion and caring towards the patient, demonstrating that the error has been taken seriously.

Further reading

Fukada, M (2018) Nursing competency: Definition, structure and development. *Journal of Medical Sciences*. Available at doi: 10.33160/yam.2018.03.001

This journal article explores definitions and attributes of nursing competency, it explains competency structure by reviewing research on the definitions.

Nursing and Midwifery Council (NMC) (2022) *An Introduction to Fitness to Practise*. Available at: www.nmc.org.uk/concerns-nurses-midwives/what-is-fitness-to-practise/an-introduction-to-fitness-to-practise/

This document is a step-by-step guide to fitness to practise. You will be able to explore the aims and objectives of the procedure and the types of cases that are considered, providing you with insight into the legal powers held by the Nursing and Midwifery Council.

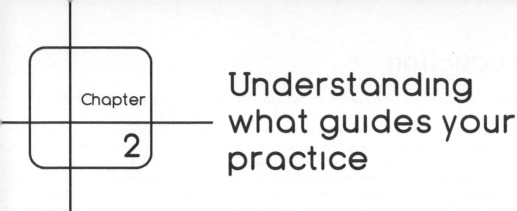

Chapter 2

Understanding what guides your practice

Chapter aims

After reading this chapter, you should be able to:

- explain terms such as ethics, morals, values and virtues and how they may influence decision making in clinical practice;
- identify key legislation relating to your role as a nursing associate;
- explore ethical and legal dilemmas and how these apply to clinical practice;
- develop critical reflection skills when presented with ethical dilemmas in clinical practice.

Introduction

As discussed in Chapter 1, nursing associates need to have awareness and knowledge around their professional behaviours to provide safe and high-quality care. This chapter will allow you to consider your own value base as you explore theories that inform ethical practice. The development of these values is critical in making important decisions in healthcare and in essence guide practice. Within the professional values of nursing practice, you will find a key focus on ethics. Ethics is a very broad subject, and, as a nursing associate, you will need to ensure that you are aware of how ethical principles influence your decision-making skills in practice. Alongside this, you will be introduced to key law and legislation which will guide your clinical decision making. By the end of the chapter you will recognise the importance of how law is used in England and Wales to protect and safeguard the people you care for. From the moment you enter healthcare you are made aware of your responsibilities and are expected to act ethically and within the law to respect the rights of the patient. This chapter will help you understand and feel confident in defining ethics and how law relates to your practice. You will be guided to do this by reflecting on practice-based studies, and applying your learning to problem solve in alternative ways. While it is acknowledged ethical practice is an essential feature of good nursing practice, what you will recognise is that at times there may not be an easy or comfortable answer to some situations. Being able to recognise and reflect on this is an important part of your learning.

Let's introduce ethics

We will begin with a quote by Socrates who stated: *the unexamined life is not worth living*. This means that you need to be reflective and occasionally question yourselves, as otherwise you will act without reason, and be unable to distinguish between good or bad actions. Working within healthcare is a moral action: what we mean by this is you need to understand your own morals and values and where these come from, to explain your actions in various situations. As a nursing associate, you will find some clinical decisions that you make will be more morally acceptable while others may not. Ethics is closely linked to your personal values and beliefs; sometimes the terms morals and ethics are used interchangeably. However, it is useful to make the following distinction: morals pertain to, or are concerned with the principles or rules of right conduct or the distinction between right and wrong (Baillie and Black, 2015). On the other side, ethics is the study of morality (morals).

Now that I have briefly introduced morals and the potential impact morals have on your ethical decision making, let's explore this concept further.

Morals: where do they come from?

Griffith and Tengnah (2020) refer to 'morals' as what a person believes is right and wrong influenced by their culture, experience, upbringing, education and religion.

Before we move on to explore what moral issues are and how they can influence your decision making when providing person-centred care, it will be useful for you to think about your moral principles.

Activity 2.1   Reflection

Earlier in the chapter the two terms ethics and morals were differentiated. Put simply, ethics was described as a system of moral principles. In clinical practice, you may come across many moral issues such as termination and euthanasia for starters that may prompt an emotional reaction. Your behaviour in these situations is guided by what you believe is 'right' and 'wrong'.

For this reflective activity, make a list of the qualities you identify as 'good' and qualities you identify as being 'bad'.

For example, you may identify telling the truth as a key quality in doing good to others.

As this activity is based on your reflection, no outline answer is provided at the end of the chapter.

Activity 2.1 encouraged you to reflect on your own moral principles and what is important to you. Now, you will have the opportunity to critically explore these moral principles in action. Moral conflict and disagreement occur frequently in healthcare practice. Given the complexity of the values that operate in healthcare, sometimes the choices you make will be 'problematic' and not shared by others or may even challenge your own moral value base.

The following case study and Activity 2.2 asks you to critically reflect on your moral principles that you identified above when presented with a moral dilemma.

Case study: Carl

Carl, a 76-year-old man, has been living in a nursing home for approximately five years. His wife Sofiya has visited him daily since he has been a resident. They have been married for nearly 60 years and Sofiya regularly tells staff that she has made it a habit to tell her husband how much she loves him whenever she sees him. Carl has instructed the staff to ensure that if his health deteriorates, his wife will be informed immediately as he wants his wife to be by his side.

One morning, Sofiya is feeling unwell and phones the residential home to specifically tell staff to share a message with Carl, saying that she loves him and will come to see him tomorrow. The nursing associate forgets to pass the message on to the nurse who is looking after Carl. Some hours later Carl asks the nurse who is looking after him if his wife has phoned and she replies that she has not. That same evening Carl's health deteriorates very rapidly. There is a delay in informing Sofiya, and she arrives later. When Sofiya arrives, Carl has already died.

The nursing associate is distressed because she did not pass Sofiya's telephone message on to Carl. When Sofiya asks the nursing associate what Carl's response was when she gave the message, the nursing associate is concerned about what to tell her.

She knows if she tells Sofiya the truth (no message was passed on) she would be very upset. Or she could lie and let her believe that the message was shared to give her solace.

Activity 2.2 Critical thinking

After reading the above case study, note down your thoughts on the following:

1. Are there any moral principles that you identified earlier that are in conflict with how you would respond in this situation?
2. What is the 'right' thing to do?
3. How can you be sure that the decisions you make and actions you take in this situation are 'morally right'?

An outline answer is provided at the end of the chapter.

This activity encouraged you to consider the issues when deciding what you believe is the right decision and best course of action to take. By doing so you have applied some key ethical principles to your moral decision making. This activity would have also highlighted situations where there might not be a single 'right' answer. It is important in such situations that you are able to discuss your decision making with a registered nurse and talk through the clinical situation.

In the next section, we will look at some ethical theories and frameworks and consider how they may apply to the case study.

Ethical theories and frameworks

There are many ethical theories and frameworks that serve as a means of providing structure to ethically sensitive situations. It is important to note these ethical structures don't always give the right answers to the moral problem. They merely support you in informing your clinical decision making and understanding why decisions or actions by yourself and/or other practitioners have been made (Harris, 2020).

Rowe et al. (2020) identifies three types of ethical enquiry, meta ethics, applied ethics and normative ethics. Normative ethics are the ethics used in healthcare. The following box will provide a summary of normative ethics.

Understanding the theory

Normative ethics are split into two types: deontology and teleology. Both of these sub-types can inform your clinical decision making in various ethically sensitive situations.

Deontology: Immanuel Kant's (1724–1804, a German philosopher) deontology theory states that the morality of an action should be based on whether that action itself is right or wrong under a series of rules, rather than based on the consequences of the action. Under duty-based ethics you cannot justify an action by showing that it produced good consequences. Relating this back to Activity 2.2, the action of the nursing associate in the situation would be to tell Sofiya the truth (which risks her being upset) but it would be wrong to tell a lie even if it meant it produced more harm (or less good) than doing the right thing.

Teleology: this theory bases its principle of whether an act is right or wrong only on the results of the act. Therefore, if you are faced with a moral dilemma the action that should be chosen is the one that maximises good consequences. In reference to Activity 2.2, if the nursing associate had to lie to Sofiya, it would be because the consequences of the mistruth would be morally relevant rather than the act of lying itself.

This theory is further broken down into three branches:

- act consequentialism;
- rules consequentialism;
- utilitarianism.

These three further branches maintain the core principles of teleology but, utilitarianism states that an action is right if it produces the greatest good for the greatest number of people, and of any two actions, the most ethical one will produce the greater balance over harms. An example of this would be the shutting down of some minority services to invest further in services that will benefit the greater number of people. An example of this can be shutting down the local youth centre as it is not frequently used to expand on an already established breast-screening service. One can argue does the mental health of youth not matter just because the service is only accessed more frequently.

The theory box provides you with a summary of the two types of normative ethics, however, within healthcare there are other theories that you need to have an awareness of. It is important as a nursing associate that you can understand the definition of these, so you are able to perform your duty with the highest regard to patient advocacy and maintain the ethics which healthcare practice is based on.

The following activity asks you to conduct research into an ethical theory called 'virtue ethics' that differs from both deontology and teleology. While virtue ethics are recognised as a form of normative ethics it is majorly contrasted to both branches.

Activity 2.3   Evidence-based practice and research

Access the resource, which is available online, *Principles of Biomedical Ethics* (Beauchamp and Childress, 2013) to gain an understanding of the Six Fundamental Virtues that Beauchamp and Childress refer to.

- Of the six virtues they refer to, is there a distinction between professional and personal virtues?
- While considering this answer refer to the *Standards of Proficiency for Nursing Associates* (2018a) and *The Code* (2018b). As a nursing associate, which of these virtues are a requisite of your professional standards?

An outline answer has been provided at the end of the chapter.

Activity 2.3 makes direct correlation between how principles of virtue ethics apply to practice, to ensure that they comply with the professional values and expectations of your role. You will now have the opportunity to explore a common approach to ethics in healthcare that was developed by Beauchamp and Childress (2013), which is based on four moral principles.

An ethical framework to ethical decision making

Beauchamp and Childress (2013) are known for their four ethical principle approach. These principles are set within a framework of biomedical ethics, meaning ethics that apply to healthcare. As it suggests, this approach is not an ethical theory but principles that underpin healthcare ethics in general and the care you deliver.

These four principles are:

- respect for autonomy – *the right to make a choice;*
- non-maleficence – *to do no harm;*
- beneficence– *to do good;*
- justice – *fair treatment.*

To apply these principles in practice, consider the following case study. Once you have read the case study you will be encouraged to critically apply your learning of the principles to justify how you would address the ethical dilemma in clinical practice.

Case study: Zara

Zara is 45 years old and has a diagnosis of autism. She has been readmitted into hospital following complications from her recent laparoscopy surgery for rectovaginal endometriosis. Zara gives a history of faecal incontinence and bleeding since discharge. Upon examination and a transvaginal ultrasound the consultant suggests surgery to repair the rectovaginal fistula. If left untreated it will cause further complications and discomfort to Zara. Zara refuses to have a needle inserted for the anaesthetic as she has a fear of needles and believes it is unfair she has to go through surgery again so soon.

The consultant is concerned if the fistula is left untreated it may become infected and be life-threatening.

Zara is accompanied by her daughter who is adamant that she should receive the treatment.

Should surgery be performed despite Zara's objections? What are your thoughts? Is your perspective weighing on deontology or teleology?

Using the above case study, we will now consider the ethical issues present using the four principles framework. The principle of autonomy has been provided as an example below, so you are able to follow the same structure to complete the remaining three principles in Activity 2.4. It is important to emphasise that the framework does not instruct you on what to do, but rather provides you with guidance to understand the issues present.

Respect for autonomy: This principle requires respect for the choice made by the individual without interference from others. In this case study Zara may not be fully autonomous (and not legally competent to refuse treatment) but this does not mean that ethically her views should not be considered and respected. She has expressed her wish of not having the needle inserted for anaesthesia; this is an expression of her autonomy. Griffith and Tengnah (2020) state in the healthcare context a patient has the right to make a decision about their care even if the refusal leads to harm or even death (principle of non-maleficence can be argued here). Yet, saying this is an autonomous decision does not have to be the 'correct' decision from an objective point of view otherwise Zara's needs and values would not be respected. However, an autonomous decision needs to be informed. Has Zara been given all available information to be able to make this informed decision?

The other dilemma to consider is whether to respect Zara's autonomy or to ignore her wishes by giving in to the demands of her daughter.

This brief critical discussion in relation to the principle of respecting autonomy and how it applies to the ethical dilemma will now allow you to complete the following activity which is designed to develop your critical thinking and decision-making abilities.

Activity 2.4   Decision making

Referring to the definitions outlined earlier in the chapter, provide a discussion of the following three principles in relation to the case study. This discussion should include your understanding of the principles in action:

- non-maleficence (must do no harm intentionally);
- beneficence (an action should promote good);
- justice (actions are fair to those involved).

An outline answer is provided at the end of the chapter.

Activity 2.4 demonstrates the complexities of clinical decision making when applying the four ethical principles. As a nursing associate you should always be guided by *The Code* (NMC, 2018b) which determines the professional and ethical values of the profession. As a nursing associate you have an ethical and professional obligation to provide overall benefit to patients with minimal harm (i.e. beneficence with non-maleficence), while maintaining the principle of autonomy when providing patient-centred care. However, as you may have identified while completing Activity 2.4, there are other factors that need to be considered when making ethical clinical decisions in the best interests of the patient. Ethical decision making is not undertaken in a vacuum.

You will now have the opportunity to explore this fundamental aspect of what guides your practice.

Introduction to law

The law is a fundamental part of nursing that underpins your relationship with society, the profession and your patients. Outcome 1.2 in the *Standards of Proficiencies for Nursing Associates* (NMC, 2018a) clearly stipulates the requirement of the nursing associate to understand and apply relevant legal requirements to all areas of practice. Similarly *The Code* (NMC, 2018b) sets out the standards for professional practice which is underpinned by law. To be able to uphold these standards you must be able to define and apply how law relates to your practice.

Law is described as: *the system of rules which a particular country or community recognises as regulating the actions of its members and which it may enforce by the imposition of penalties* (Oxford English Dictionary, 2021).

The law of the United Kingdom is split into three legal systems: England and Wales, Northern Ireland and Scotland, with each having its own legal system. Before you have the opportunity to explore the types of law there are, have an attempt at completing the following activity.

Activity 2.5   Reflection

Functions of law in healthcare practice
Before reading on, make a list of the functions you think law has in nursing practice.
An outline answer is provided at the end of the chapter.

Activity 2.5 encourages you to think about the role of law in healthcare practice. While undertaking this activity you may or may not have explored your role as a trainee nursing associate and the recognition that you are expected to live up to the standards of *The Code* (NMC, 2018b) and the law during your training as well. Chapter 1 discussed the accountable practitioner and if as a trainee nursing associate, your behaviours fall below the standards required, you are held accountable in line with the fitness to practise guidance published by the Nursing and Midwifery Council as well as to patients, colleagues and your employer.

Types of law

The legal system is split into two types of law: criminal and civil law.

Criminal law – refers to a body of laws that apply to criminal acts. These acts are concerned with that which is damaging socially. In healthcare practice, some of these criminal activities can include theft from a patient, murder, manslaughter or assault of a patient.

Civil law – is concerned with civil wrongs which are referred to as actions in 'tort'. In tort law a person's legal right must have been breached (most notably acts of negligence which include breach of confidentiality or failure to gain consent) and disputes can occur between individuals, organisations or between two organisations. This type of dispute usually results in compensation awarded to the 'claimant'.

The courts of England and Wales are headed by Senior Courts of England, which consist of the Courts of Appeal, the High Court of Justice (for civil cases) and the Crown Court (for criminal cases).

How are laws created?

Laws are created by Parliament; a new law or bill is considered by the House of Commons, and appointed by the House of Lords before receiving royal assent by the sovereign and becoming an Act of Parliament. The journey before an Act becomes an Act of Parliament starts off as a proposed bill. A bill is a proposal for a new law or amendment to an existing law. Not all bills that are proposed become Acts of Parliament. In terms of nursing practice, you will find law determined by statute, which means it is found in legislation and therefore is set by Parliament. You may also have heard of common law, also known as case law, which may have an impact on practice. These are laws that have been created following a legal case which has become legislation.

Now that you have been given a brief introduction of how laws are created, it might also be useful for your professional development to research these further to gain a deeper understanding. A useful resource to obtain relevant understanding is the Government website www.legislation. gov.uk. This website will also provide you with relevant information about the changes to UK law following its departure from the European Union.

As previously mentioned, law is determined by statute, which is found in legislation. The following activity will enable you to explore some of the common statute law (known as Acts) relevant to your role as a nursing associate. The Acts that are relevant in healthcare are referred to as public general Acts.

Activity 2.6   Reflection

Reflect and make a list of the Acts that you are aware of that are used in your field of nursing. As nursing associates are not field specific, are you aware of other Acts that are used in other fields of nursing? To help you with this activity and engage in peer discussion, this activity can also be undertaken in small groups.

This activity will later support you in the chapter when you focus on specific Acts that are relevant to nursing associate practice.

As this activity is based on your own reflection, no outline answer is provided at the end of the chapter.

Completing Activity 2.6 would have illustrated the Acts that are used in healthcare practice and guide your clinical decision making. You may have recognised some Acts which are used across all four fields of nursing and some which may only be used in specific fields. Some Acts that are relevant to nursing associate practice are as follows:

*   The Human Rights Act (1998);
*   Mental Capacity (Amendment) Act 2019;
*   The Mental Health Act (1983 amended in 2007);
*   Children Act (1989);
*   Equality Act (2010);
*   Health and Social Care Act (2012).

This is by no means a comprehensive list of Acts that are used in clinical practice to inform clinical decision making. Healthcare practitioners are guided by other Acts when making clinical decisions – an example of this is the Abortion Act 1967. While as a nursing associate, you will not be authorising an abortion, you may be involved in providing care for a woman who is. Therefore, working within your scope of practice and having an understanding that Acts are not limited to the above will provide you with an awareness when working across different specialities. The next section will allow you to develop and apply your application of knowledge of the above legislation to clinical scenarios.

Applying legislation in practice

This section of the chapter has been written in smaller paragraphs and sub-divided into the four fields of nursing to enable you to apply relevant legislation for each field of nursing. There will be instances whereby more than one of the above legislation will apply to a case scenario. It is your opportunity to develop your critical thinking and analysis when engaging in the activities.

Paediatrics

We recommend that you read the initial scenario and suggested questions, and then consider the relevant issues and what action you might take. You are required to read and research the Children Act (1989) and the Human Rights Act (1998). You can find the weblink to both acts in the annotated further reading section at the end of the chapter.

Case study: *Gard and Others v. the United Kingdom* (2017)

The Charlie Gard case was a best interests case in 2017 involving Charles Matthew William Gard, born with mitochondrial DNA depletion syndrome (MDDS), a rare genetic disorder that causes progressive brain damage and muscle failure. MDDS has no treatment and usually causes death in infancy. The case became controversial because the medical team and parents disagreed about whether experimental treatment was in the best interests of the child.

Charlie was placed on mechanical ventilation and MDDS was diagnosed. Experimental treatment was agreed between the hospital and the neurologist based in New York. In January, after Charlie had seizures that caused brain damage, the hospital trust formed the view that further treatment was futile and might prolong suffering. They began discussions with the parents about ending life support and providing palliative care.

Charlie's parents still wanted to try the experimental treatment and raised funds for a transfer to a hospital in New York. In February 2017 the hospital trust asked the High Court to override the parents' decision, questioning the potential of nucleoside therapy to treat Charlie's condition. On 27 July, by consent, Charlie was transferred to a hospice, mechanical ventilation was withdrawn, and he died the next day at the age of 11 months and 24 days.

Activity 2.7　Evidence-based practice and research

After reading the above case study, consider the following questions:

1. What rights do parents have to determine treatment?
2. Which principles of the Children Act (1989) were particularly relevant in this case?
3. Which articles from the Human Rights Act (1998) may be relevant here that can be argued are being denied?

An outline answer is provided at the end of the chapter.

Activity 2.7 should have provided you with an understanding of the Children Act (1989), which relates to children and young people under the age of 18 addressing family law. It is particularly relevant to your role as a nursing associate as it allocates duties to local authorities, courts, parents and health and social care organisations to ensure children are safeguarded and their welfare is promoted. It is imperative to note that while researching into the Act, you may have come across an amendment to the Act titled Children Act 2004, largely in consequence to the Victoria Climbie inquiry. As a nursing associate you need to be aware amendments are made to Acts and it is your responsibility to keep your professional development up to date.

The following case study has been intended to provoke thought and discussion with respect to issues pertaining to learning disabilities and the mental health field of nursing. Both of these fields of nursing will be explored separately but the same case study used to develop your critical thinking.

Case study: Reeyah

You are a nursing associate employed on the Sunrise Ward managed by the local mental health NHS trust. Reeyah, a 31-year-old Indian woman, has been admitted to the ward following a physical assault by her carer who is also a sibling. She was removed by the community mental health team as she lacked capacity to decide where to live. She has complex needs, she is mildly deaf with a diagnosis of bipolar disorder and Down's syndrome. A Deprivation of Liberty Safeguards was authorised by the NHS trust under the Mental Capacity Act 2005 a month after she had arrived at the ward. The authorisation lapsed. A solicitor on behalf of Reeyah's family contended that the current arrangements amount to a deprivation of liberty and that there should no longer be a reason for lawful authorisation for her deprivation of liberty. Reeyah has engaged with her treatment and is taking her medication on time. She is happy and has made no attempts to leave.

You will now have the opportunity to explore the learning disabilities field of healthcare and some of the prominent legislation active when caring for those within this field.

Learning disabilities

A learning disability has been described by the World Health Organization (2021) as an *impairment of skills which contributes to the overall level of intelligence, i.e. cognitive, language, motor and social abilities*. In your practice as a nursing associate it is imperative that you are aware of the laws that protect and safeguard vulnerable adults in your care. *The Code* (NMC, 2018b) emphasises the importance of upholding and respecting the human rights of those you care for. Some of the laws that will guide your practice for vulnerable adults include the Human Rights Act (1998), The Mental Capacity Act (2005) and The Mental Health Act (1983).

The Mental Capacity Act (2005) is law to all health and social care workers. Its legal framework is there to enable and safeguard people over the age of 16 who may be unable to make decisions: in such cases a best interests decision must be made for them. It also gives legal protection to the health professionals who care for them.

Some reasons why someone may lack capacity:

- severe learning disability;
- effects of alcohol, illegal drugs and prescription medication;
- dementia;
- head injury;
- stroke.

This is not a comprehensive list. The main principles of the Mental Capacity Act 2005 should be followed when consent is obtained for treatment. The following principles apply for the purposes of this Act.

- A person must be assumed to have capacity unless it is established that they lack capacity.
- A person is not to be treated as unable to make a decision unless all practicable steps to help them to do so have been taken without success.
- A person is not to be treated as unable to make a decision merely because they make an unwise decision.
- An act done, or decision made, under this Act for or on behalf of a person who lacks capacity must be done, or made, in their best interests.

- Before the act is done, or the decision is made, regard must be had to whether the purpose for which it is needed can be as effectively achieved in a way that is less restrictive of the person's rights and freedom of action.

(DoH 2021)

Capacity refers to the ability to make a particular decision at a particular time. It is wrong to refer to a person as having or lacking capacity for all decisions. If an individual lacks capacity to consent to their care and treatment, for their own protection they may be deprived of their liberty. For the following activity, Deprivation of Liberty Safeguards will be explored.

Activity 2.8   Critical thinking

The Deprivation of Liberty Safeguards (DoLS), which only apply to England and Wales, are an amendment to the Mental Capacity Act 2005. This was a response to a European Court of Human Rights ruling that a man who lacked decision-making capacity had been detained in hospital against his wishes *(HL v United Kingdom (45508/99), 2005)*. The DoLS under the MCA allows restraint and restrictions that amount to a deprivation of liberty to be used in hospitals and care homes – but only if they are in a person's best interests. To deprive a person of their liberty, care homes and hospitals must request standard authorisation from a local authority. In July 2018, the government published a bill, which passed law in May 2019 to replace DoLS with a scheme to be known as Liberty Protection Safeguards. However, this scheme will be implemented on 1 April 2022.

There are six assessments which have to take place before a standard authorisation can be given for someone to be deprived of their liberty. Article 5 of the Human Rights Act (1998) states *everyone has the right to liberty and security of person. No one shall be deprived of his or her liberty (unless) in accordance with a procedure prescribed in law.* The six assessments is a procedure prescribed in law. You can read more around the six assessments on the Social Care Institute for Excellence from the following link www.scie.org.uk/mca/imca/roles/assessments.

Now refer to the case study and answer the following questions. I would encourage you to initiate these discussions with your practice assessor who may be able to provide you with further information when making informed decisions when answering the questions.

1. Considering the Mental Capacity Act 2005 and the DoLS directive, what factors would need to be considered to authorise a deprivation of liberty for Reeyah again?
2. From your personal reflection, do you think she meets the criteria? Access the above resource for support in answering this question if required.

An outline answer is provided at the end of the chapter.

This activity would have initiated a discussion around the issues present when protecting the human rights of vulnerable people who may lack capacity to make certain decisions. Vulnerable adults are protected under the Mental Capacity Act 2005, however, this is not the only law that protects vulnerable people. Read on to learn how those patients with mental disorders are protected.

Mental health

The Mental Health Act 1983 is the law in England and Wales. It was updated in 2007. Divided up into ten parts, it informs of the rights of people with mental disorders in respect of care and treatment. The Mental Health Act 2007 amendment saw several definitions of 'mental disorder' omitted. A mental disorder has been described as any disorder or disability of the mind (Mental Health Act 1983). You may have heard of the word 'sectioning'; what this means under the Mental Health Act 1983 is that people can be detained in hospital under a section of the Mental Health Act, and are therefore not free to leave. The Act covers the rights of patients when they have been detained against their wishes amongst other rights. It should not be assumed those with learning disabilities are suffering from a mental disorder and can be detained formally unless that disability is associated with abnormally aggressive or serious conduct. More information can be explored about the Mental Health Act 1983 at www. legislation.gov.uk.

Activity 2.9   Reflection

Refer to the case study on Reeyah and answer the following question.

- Why is Reeyah not detainable under the Mental Health Act 1983?

An outline answer is provided at the end of the chapter.

Activity 2.9 illustrates how more than one law can be utilised to protect patients' rights while in your care. It is your responsibility to have an understanding of these so you are able to promote person-centred care.. The Equality Act 2010 is another piece of legislation that legally safeguards people from discrimination. The following activity has been provided for you to critically explore how this law can be applied in the following case study.

Case study: Julie and Tina

Julie and Tina, a same-sex couple, were refused access to fertility treatment on the NHS as they did not meet the necessary criteria to receive NHS-funded treatment. They were eventually allowed to have fertility treatment on the NHS after their local health authority accepted that to deny them access to treatment would be discriminative.

If you explore the above situation, it raises many questions regarding how the couple's human rights as well as their protected characteristics, which are legally protected under the Equality Act 2010, were unfairly discriminated against. Now turn your attention to Activity 2.10.

Activity 2.10   Critical thinking

As a nursing associate you are required to discuss the type of discrimination encountered and under which protected characteristics this discrimination was encountered.

To be able to support you with completing this activity refer to www.legislation.gov.uk, which will provide you with information around the legislation.

An outline answer is provided at the end of the chapter.

The Equality Act 2010 will affect your clinical practice frequently and to be able to recognise the types of discrimination as well as the nine protected characteristics will enable you to identify situations when people are being unfairly discriminated against and what your duty in that situation is. You may have also come across the term 'postcode lottery' in the NHS. This term is shorthand for random countrywide variations in the provision and quality of public services. Where you live will define the type of service you can expect. Does this count as discriminatory practice? An example of the postcode lottery can be seen applied to the number of IVF cycles an individual can have, which depends on geographical location. Is this fair? The following link will provide you with further information around access to IVF treatment: www.nice.org.uk/news/article/nice-calls-for-an-end-to-postcode-lottery-of-ivf-treatment

Your professional duties as a nursing associate are guided by professional standards and by now you will have identified the importance of how law and ethics inform clinical decision making to uphold the principles of person-centred care.

Chapter summary

This chapter has provided you with an introduction to how ethical theories/frameworks and relevant law apply to your clinical practice. As a nursing associate the opportunity to work across the four fields of nursing brings the unique opportunity for you to explore how legislation is applied to specific fields of nursing. Yet, while critically discussing the activities provided, you should have also recognised key legislation is applicable to most areas of practice and usually more than one key legislation is used to protect and safeguard the rights of the people in your care. Importantly, as part of your continual professional development and being able to use current evidence-based practice in clinical decision making, you are reminded that laws and ethical knowledge need to be kept up to date if you are to uphold the standards that govern your practice. Further reading web resources have been provided throughout the chapter enabling you to implement these in your evidence-based research discussions, yet you are also guided to work within your scope of practice which means liaising with line managers and registered nurses when you are presented with practice dilemmas you are unsure of. This is particularly relevant when presented with ethical dilemmas that may require reflection or clinical supervision. Doing so will ensure you are practising in a safe and effective manner that upholds the principles of person-centred care.

Activities: Brief outline answers

Activity 2.2 Critical thinking (page 26)

You may have considered some of the following issues that have emerged from the activity.

1. Are there any moral principles that you identified earlier that are in conflict with how you would respond in this situation?

You may have identified telling the truth and being honest at all times as a moral principle that is important to you. But this may have been challenged, for example, while you may believe that the wife has a right to be told the truth whatever the circumstance and it is your duty to tell the truth. You may also be conflicted and consider that the truth will hurt her deeply and may cause her considerable upset. You may believe you have a duty not to hurt her and ensure her happiness in this situation.

2. What is the 'right' thing to do?

This will be largely based on consequence. The consequence of being truthful or lying to the wife. Would the wife lose trust in you and the healthcare profession if she found out you had lied to her. The right thing to do in this situation will be influenced by factors such as your culture, your upbringing, your experience or your religion. You may consider the moral principle of treating others the way you want to be treated which has roots in religious teaching. This will allow you to think about the situation they are in instead of just your own.

3. How can you be sure that the decisions you make and actions you take in this situation are 'morally right'?

You can consider what you would want someone to do for you if you were in that situation.

Activity 2.3 Evidence-based practice and research (page 27)

Summary of the Six Fundamental Virtues:

- care;
- compassion;discernment;
- trustworthiness;
- integrity;
- conscientiousness.

These Six Fundamental Virtues are fundamentally the essence of your professional virtues as indicated in your professional standards and ethical Code of Practice .

Activity 2.4 Decision making (page 29)

Non-maleficence – As a moral principle this means do no harm, meaning not injuring or causing harm to others. Zara would be harmed if she was forcibly restrained to have the needle inserted for the anaesthesia. However, if she was not treated there is the risk that she may develop an infection which could be life-threatening. Which course of action would result in the greatest harm? This assessment relies on assumptions: how successful will the operation be for Zara as this will be her second surgery? How likely is it that Zara will be readmitted again for complications if she does not have surgery?

As a nursing associate you have a duty to act in the best interests of the patient as stipulated in *The Code* (NMC, 2018b). This principle can be overridden by the principle of beneficence, doing good in the longer term.

Beneficence– A nursing associate should act to benefit their patients; this may clash with the principle of respecting the patient's autonomy. What needs to be considered here is the long- and short-term effects of overriding Zara's views. In the short term the insertion of the needle for anaesthesia may cause emotional distress and pain from this action. However, overriding her wish will be of benefit for the long term as without treatment she will suffer serious long-term health implications that may be life-threatening. The benefits must outweigh the implications of not overriding her request (from a legal perspective a competent person's wishes cannot be overridden in their best interests).

Justice – This principle is based on an obligation to treat others fairly. Treating others fairly means to act justly and that is to give them what is theirs rightfully. Equal access to services should be given regardless of race, gender, socioeconomic status or religion. In relation to the case study, it would be relevant to consider the cost effectiveness of the treatment options and the impact the decision about her treatment has on resources available to others.

Activity 2.5 Reflection (page 30)

Functions of law in nursing practice:

- protects patients' rights;
- imposes minimum standards of acceptable care and behaviour as a registered professional;
- maintains a standard of nursing practice, which makes nursing associates accountable;
- differentiates between responsibilities which are different from other healthcare professionals.

Activity 2.7 Evidence-based practice and research (page 32)

1. When parents do not agree about a child's future treatment, it is a standard legal process to ask the courts to make a decision. Parents have a central role in decision making (Children Act 1989 – Article 1 Welfare of the Child). Their wishes are not conclusive and can be overruled. They do not have a legal right to insist that treatment is withdrawn or insisted. They should be given clear information about treatment options, likely outcomes and prognosis.

2. The principles and provisions of the Children Act 1989 that are particularly relevant to this case are:
    - the definitions of parental rights and responsibilities;
    - the paramountcy and the definition of the child's best interests;
    - the 'no order' principle and;
    - the 'no delay' principle.

3. Under Article 2 (right to life) that the hospital has blocked access to life-sustaining treatment (in the USA) for Charlie and under Article 5 (right to liberty and security) that, as a result, he is unlawfully deprived of his liberty. Articles 6 (right to a fair trial) and 8 (right to respect for private and family life) that the domestic court decisions amounted to an unfair and disproportionate interference in their parental rights.

Activity 2.8 Critical thinking (page 34)

Reeyah would need to meet the six assessment criteria which includes the following:

- mental capacity;
- best interest;
- no refusals;
- eligibility;
- mental health;
- age.

Activity 2.9 Reflection (page 35)

Reeyah is not detainable under the Mental Health Act 1983 because she does not meet the criteria. Her learning disability does not mean she is incapable of making an informed decision. She is complying with treatment and does not demonstrate any behaviours to imply she needs involuntary detainment. If Reeyah's liberties were deprived then this would be through an assessment with the DoLs directive under the Mental Health Act 1983.

Activity 2.10 Critical thinking (page 36)

What type of discrimination did the couple encounter?

- direct discrimination – this occurs where a health service treats someone less favourably because of one or more protected characteristics.

Under which protected characteristic was this discrimination encountered?

- sexual orientation.

Further reading

Beauchamp, T and Childress, J (2013) *Principles of Biomedical Ethics.* 7th edition. Oxford: Oxford University Press.

This book is one of the most important and influential books in the field of bioethics. It is commonly referred to in nursing practice.

Griffith, R and Tengnah, C (2020) *Law and Professional Issues in Nursing.* 5th edition. London: SAGE.

This book provides case studies which encourage reflective and critical discussion skills in relation to law in nursing practice. It is mapped to the 2018 NMC standards allowing you to understand how the discussions relate to practice.

Harris, M (2020) *Understanding Person-Centred Care for Nursing Associates*. London: SAGE.

This book has been written primarily for nursing associates. It covers topics related to providing evidence-based person-centred care. With activities ranging from critical discussion, reflection and use of evidence-based practice in research it is a great addition to your understanding of the nursing associate role.

Useful websites

www.scie.org.uk/mca/imca/roles/assessments

Social Care Institute for Excellence (2021) Mental Capacity Act (MCA) IMCAs and assessments.

Visit this webpage which takes you to the six assessments required of the patient for a DoLs standard authorisation to be satisfied.

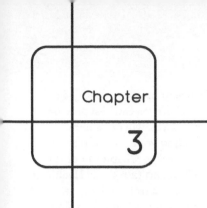

Chapter

3

The interdisciplinary team and how its members influence care

Chapter aims

After reading this chapter, you should be able to:

* understand the role of interdisciplinary teams in care of complex patient needs;
* understand how your role is integrated within interdisciplinary teams;
* understand and respect diversity in the wider health and social care teams.

Introduction

Understanding your role and responsibilities is an essential part of developing your identity as a nursing associate. It will help you to recognise limitations of your role and how you can best provide high quality of care to patients. However, for patient care to be successful, you will be required to work within complex teams on a daily basis, therefore only understanding your own role is not enough. To revisit the background of NA role development, please refer back to Chapter 1 or look at the additional resources at the end of the chapter, to access the Francis Report (2013) and Health Education England website. This chapter will introduce you to a concept of 'interdisciplinary team working' and the different members that make up a team. Following this chapter, you will explore further tools and skills that you can use and develop your role within a team. Teams can be very complex and vary from setting to setting, especially in healthcare. This means that understanding how your role fits in can be a difficult task to achieve. Nevertheless, teamwork and effective communication within them has been identified as a significant factor contributing to better patient outcomes, patient satisfaction and reduced number of errors (Robson, 2017). This makes it a priority for you to understand how teams work most effectively and your own role within them.

If you searched for the term 'nursing associate role in teams', you would probably not get many suggestions to follow up on. This is because the NA role is new and will require further evidence-based research to evaluate its exact role and how it best fits teams in a variety of healthcare settings. It will also look very different, depending on what field or speciality you come from (or have joined recently). This means that you will need to use general principles discussed in this chapter to reflect on what your role is as an individual professional and a team member. This not a disadvantage, but rather a very unique position to make positive changes in healthcare team dynamics, ultimately, positively affecting the quality of patient care.

Below is a direct quote from a qualified nursing associate, who is sharing some examples of the positive impact their role has on practice.

> *The training and education that I have received in becoming a registered nursing associate has helped be to become a caring professional. I work in a Special Needs school, where the majority of the students have complex health conditions. Most of the students are non-verbal and this is why I feel it is imperative to maintain high standards of care, dignity and compassion. Although these children cannot vocalise their feelings of pain, they are able to express these emotions through their body language. This is how I feel I make the most impact, by being considerate to their needs and requirements. It is important to get to know your patients, in my case students, and look out for cues that may indicate feelings. I feel the importance of introducing myself and talking through interaction with them cannot be underestimated, as they cannot read my name badge or ask any questions. Over time I have noticed the smiles and positive cues, which give me an immense satisfaction that I am delivering person-centred care to the best of my ability as a nursing associate.*

This chapter will introduce you to Alma, who started her nursing associate training programme, after being a healthcare assistant on the same acute medicine ward for over ten years. Alma was faced with multiple challenges in becoming a TNA, mostly related to feelings of 'belonging' on her own ward. Alma's scenario demonstrates the importance of good leadership and guidance within a team, especially when new members join a team and affect the dynamics of an already formed team.

While every team you work within will be different, there are key factors which can be identified as essential within every single team. Having a shared goal within a team enables all individuals to stay focused and determined, while also remaining motivated and satisfied within their job roles. However, working within a multidisciplinary team means that every professional has their own agenda when it comes to patient care. The literature has therefore recently focused more on emphasising the importance of working as an interdisciplinary team rather than a multidisciplinary team. For example, Health Education England (HEE) (2021) have recently published a toolkit on 'Working differently together', which aims to support building teams who work together towards providing excellent patient care. We will therefore look further into the meaning behind these terms and what it means to you as a TNA or NA in practice.

Teamwork amongst nursing associates

It is important to acknowledge that although nursing associates are now working within wider existing teams, they are also learning how to work together. This can be a complex task, due to a range of practitioners, from a variety of fields of nursing, who are trained to become general nursing associates, with knowledge on all fields of healthcare practice.

If you reflect on your own background and job experience, you can probably identify multiple teams that you have been part of; these may be within a healthcare setting or other industries. Teamwork is not a new concept and is integrated within many industries to reach better outcomes and profit organisations. However, there is a smaller chance that you have worked within a completely newly formed team, where your and your colleagues' roles are still being identified and are evolving. This may be even more complex due to the background of nursing associates, whose original field of nursing may be adult, children's, mental health or learning disabilities, especially if you all now work within a field of nursing that is new to the majority of the team. Finding the shared goal becomes difficult, as you may all have different priorities in care.

This is where good leadership and education is an essential characteristic of the team. A good leader should be able to clearly identify everyone's role within teams and collaborate within the interdisciplinary team to ensure effectiveness and shared purpose (Barr and Dowding, 2019). Therefore, for example, instead of just prioritising patients' mental health needs, you can work together to create a plan, which holistically benefits the patient and also takes your strengths into consideration.

Interdisciplinary team

To understand how a team works together, you first need to understand what we mean by interdisciplinary teams. But before we get there, let's have a closer look at what we mean by teamwork.

Defining teamwork

A team is made up of individuals who are working towards a shared goal or an outcome (Ryan, 2017). In healthcare, this usually relates to a multidisciplinary team who are working towards a goal of positively affecting patient outcomes, and individuals are professionals within their fields of health and social care. Good teamwork practices in healthcare can have positive effects on patient safety, patient outcomes and also staff job satisfaction (Gluyas, 2015). When considering the shared goals that teams are aiming for, this usually relates to complex patient needs, which require input from a variety of professionals. If the goal that each professional had was not a shared one, but based on the specific need of that patient, this could result in breakdown of communication and even possible harm to the patient. Due to patients requiring treatment plans for multiple conditions, a number of health and social care professionals need to be involved. Although professionals are able to provide good-quality care alone, they are likely to need specialist input from others. This could be a very narrow view on the care plan, as multiple professionals working together to improve a patient's condition would lead to a better outcome. For example, while a general practitioner (GP) has been trained in many different conditions and has many skills to assess patients across a lifespan (from pre-conception to older patients), they continue to closely liaise with specialist consultants and other services to make appropriate referrals to enhance care quality. This does not mean that the GP is not confident in their skills or abilities, but rather has self-awareness of their own limitations of practice, which brings patients' care and safety as a priority. This way, teams can work well together, by recognising individual strengths and weaknesses.

So what makes a good team? There are many individuals working within health and social care settings, who come from a variety of backgrounds professionally and personally. For the team to work well together, it is not enough to understand what their common goal is. Other characteristics, such as being approachable, willing to compromise, being dedicated to their task and assertiveness, have to be considered and maintained. Of course, this is not an exhaustive list and is evolving, depending on the team and its needs (Campbell, 2020).

Platform 4, within *Nursing Associate Proficiency Standards*, focuses on expectations of NAs while working in teams (NMC, 2018a). It provides clear goals for your development, as by the end of your training to become a qualified NA, you must meet each of these standards. Some of these might seem obvious to you, while others may require further discussion with your practice supervisors and colleagues.

Activity 3.1 Reflective and critical thinking

- What do you think makes up a good team? List as many characteristics as you can think of.
- Does your team match these attributes?
- If not, what is missing and why?

As this activity is based on your own reflection, no outline answer is provided at the end of this chapter.

This activity aims to establish what you already know about the importance and effectiveness of a good team. It is easy to think of only yourself, your own role and responsibilities, however, chances are that you have already worked or will be working in teams that are carefully organised and chosen, to enable collaborative working.

How do teams form?

In healthcare, teams form for many different reasons and can be very small, consisting of only a few professionals or can be very large, such as found on a specialist ward. Both team sizes have advantages and disadvantages; for example, a smaller team may find it easier to keep up with communication and have more time to get to know one another's strengths and weaknesses. However, if there are personality or value clashes within that team, the effects of conflict can have a major disruption to their performance, if not resolved quickly by the leader. On the other hand, larger teams may find it difficult to keep up to date with one another and effective communication may be difficult to always achieve; however, it may be easier for the leader to navigate personality differences or other issues without affecting the team's performance. One thing that any team does have to go through, however, is the initial forming stage when a new team is created. This may make you feel better as a NA, as your role is new to most teams at this current moment or it may make you feel nervous, as you will need to settle into an already formed team. Joining a new team will always have its challenges, no matter if your role is new or already established and it is useful to remember that all teams constantly go through changes in group dynamics.

There are many different theories and models used in literature and practice to help understand how teams work. All of them have their own strengths and weaknesses, therefore the organiser or leader of the team has to carefully consider which approach to use within their team. One of the commonly applied theories has been developed by Bruce Tuckman in 1965, who initially came up with four stages of team development: forming, storming, norming and performing (Tuckman, 1965). The first stage of forming includes the team members being brought together and getting to know one another's strengths and weaknesses; at this stage, no one is really sure of who is responsible for what or what the shared goal within the team is. Next up is storming, where conflict may arise and individual personality types may become apparent. This is the stage where the team is slightly unsettled; however, start the communication process and develop clarity about the hierarchy. If this stage is managed successfully by the leader, it usually leads to great progress in team dynamics, as clear roles and responsibilities emerge and team members start working well together. This is called the norming stage. Finally, this leads to the team being able to make actual progress towards reaching the shared goal, and effective communication is achieved during the performing stage. Later, the adjourning stage was added to the theory, as once the task has been completed, there is a sense of achievement reached.

This theory helps to describe how some teams form; however, it is important to highlight that it is not a set scenario. Many variables can be presented within the team, meaning that the team will move back and forwards between the different stages until they reach the 'performing' stage and produce real output. This is completely normal and the reason why commitment to your own role and communication will aid you in settling in within a new team.

Please see the further reading section at the end of this chapter for examples of other teamwork theories that will help you to develop further understanding of how teams form and develop, especially within healthcare. Don't forget to consider barriers and challenges teams may face when implementing any teamwork theory. This will help you to develop critical thinking while reading new information, which is an essential skill for NAs within academia and practice.

Collaborative approach to patient care

Now that we have discussed what we mean by teamwork and multidisciplinary teams, we can discuss interdisciplinary team working. Although they sound very similar, there are some key differences between them which you need to be aware of as a NA.

Consider the case study below, which demonstrates a team of professionals working together towards providing support for one patient's recovery.

Case study: Jonathan

Jonathan (21 years old) suffered a stroke six months ago, due to haemorrhagic stroke. This has left him with severe right-sided body weakness, dysphasia (slurred speech) and difficulty swallowing. He has now been discharged from hospital and is continuing his recovery in the community. His mum is his carer at the moment, although Jonathan is hoping to make a good recovery so that he can continue his plans to go to university and study chemical engineering.

(**Further reading opportunity**: Access the National Institute for Health and Care Excellence (NICE) guidelines on managing intracerebral haemorrhage, to develop

(Continued)

(Continued)

understanding on managing the acute stage of this condition. A link to the guidelines is available in the further reading section, at the end of this chapter).

Since then, his recovery has been very complex and challenging, requiring many different professionals to be involved in his care. Jonathan's mother has a folder with copies of his care plans for recovery and there are four different ones at the moment.

- Physiotherapy: Jonathan attends a physiotherapy appointment once a week at his local hospital, to assess his progress and they provide him with exercises to do until the next appointment. Jonathan must practise the exercises in order to strengthen his muscles and make progress with his mobility.
- Occupation therapy: Jonathan attends occupation therapy appointment once every week to practise essential skills, such as washing and dressing himself, pouring a drink and generally using equipment around him.
- Speech and language therapy (SALT): currently, Jonathan sees someone from SALT once every two weeks to reassess his swallowing, speech and set exercises for the next two weeks.
- Stroke specialist nurse: appointments scheduled every three months to review overall progress. Jonathan's mum tends to always come to these appointments, so that she is aware of any changes in the rehabilitation plan.
- The stroke specialist nurse regularly checks in with each of the other healthcare professionals involved in the care and reviews progress that Jonathan has made so far. This is done by reading regular reports on care plan progress. Recently, it has become apparent that Jonathan is not progressing very well with each of the professionals and has missed a few appointments. This, unfortunately, was not picked up for four months and has therefore delayed Jonathan's recovery, as he hasn't progressed within his care plan goals. His mother was not aware of any issues, as she hasn't been attending all the appointments and Jonathan has not communicated with anyone about this either.

Williams et al. (2019) highlight that stroke rehabilitation should be priority amongst all healthcare professionals involved within care and it should be goal orientated, which are set by the patients themselves with the support of the MDT. What has happened above, is that each individual MDT member has carried out tasks within their specific care plans, without acknowledging the progress Jonathan has been making overall in his rehabilitation.

Activity 3.2   Scenario assessment

Consider the following points below, before continuing to read further.

1. What do you think could be the potential problem that is affecting Jonathan in engaging with his recovery plan?
2. Who else do you think should be included within this team of healthcare professionals supporting Jonathan within his recovery?
3. In what way could the team of healthcare professionals work more as an interdisciplinary team?

An outline answer for questions 1 and 2 is provided at the end of this chapter.

Let's consider the potential answer to the third question together: a multidisciplinary approach to rehabilitation is very important as highlighted previously, especially when navigating short- and long-term goals towards a patient's recovery. Each healthcare professional devises a care plan with the patient to determine the specific needs and goals and regularly reviews the progress. However, this is not enough as overall recovery depends on the progress made by the whole MDT. Therefore, close communication between the healthcare professionals on progress reviews is essential throughout each patient's recovery. Teams should meet on a regular basis to integrate all the care plans together and determine if any changes need to be made, based on other aspects of recovery. This is interdisciplinary working, as instead of healthcare professionals having their own agenda, care plans are integrated together depending on progress overall within each speciality. This not only affects the team's success, as they will be maintaining higher quality standards, but also will positively affect the patient's outcomes due to the holistic approach to care. This further reduces the risk of errors being made, which could affect patient safety and long-term recovery. Communicating via good record keeping would also be essential here to ensure accurate information is passed on between teams. Annex A, within *Standards of Proficiency for Nursing Associates*, provides a list of skills which underpin your role in communicating information to other healthcare professionals and service users (NMC, 2018a). So, while each of the individual roles are important in healthcare, we also need to be aware how well teams work together and communicate any updates to one another. This is also where understanding of your own role within a team becomes a priority, as well as understanding your colleagues' roles.

Attitude towards collaboration

You may feel confident in your own role and feel that you can do your job well by yourself. Why do you need to work so closely with other team members and get to know them? Hopefully the scenario above about Jonathan has already helped you to understand why that is important in terms of patient care. Having the positive attitude and enthusiasm to work collaboratively will naturally lead to you having more conversations with your colleagues, getting to know their roles and their personalities (Lake et al., 2015). Knowing your team's strengths and weaknesses enables you to make better decisions in practice when working together in a team. This means that you and your colleagues are able to identify the most suitable person for the job and delegate responsibilities appropriately. It can take some time to achieve such performance within the team, where everyone is aware of their strengths and communicates effectively, but having a positive attitude and a team approach helps towards this. Lake at al. (2015) further highlights that key to successful team collaboration is trust. Your colleagues should be able to trust that any tasks delegated to you will be completed to a high standard and that any issues will be communicated back. Trust can also take time to develop, therefore getting to know your colleagues, offering help when needed and recognising when someone may be feeling overwhelmed, will over time lead to team members trusting one another.

Activity 3.3   Critical thinking

Consider the diagram below, what do you think is the most important factor that contributes to collaborative working? Explain your answer.

As this activity is based on your own critical thinking, no outline answer is provided at the end of this chapter.

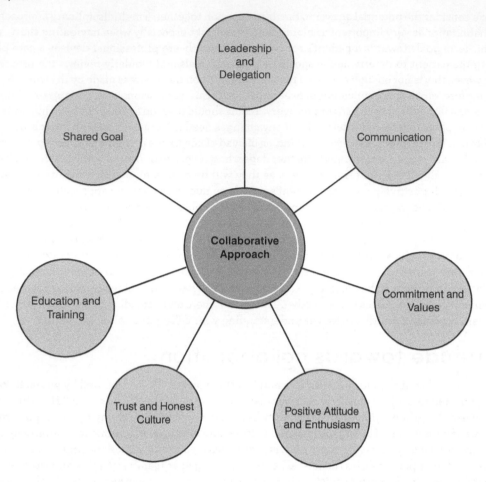

Figure 3.1 Factors contributing to collaborative approach in teams

You may have identified communication as the most important aspect of teamwork and we would agree with you. Effective communication ensures that all team members have the most recent information, enabling them to be more efficient within their roles, while also still contributing to the team's overall goal. This is especially true in healthcare, where treatment and care plans change constantly. Communicating updates means patient safety is maintained and the majority of errors are avoided due to lack of knowledge about a situation/changes. It is impossible to work together but not talk or pass over information using other methods, such as handovers or huddles. This list is certainly not exhaustive and you may be able to think of a few more factors which could contribute to an effective collaborative approach. Some differences between teams are expected, depending on the nature of the team and overall goal, however, key factors are highlighted within the diagram and are essential to any team working efficiently together.

Understanding your professional role and responsibilities already helps you towards achieving some of these collaborative approach factors within your team, as you will be guided by the *Standards of Proficiency* (NMC, 2018a) to communicate effectively, to keep up with your training, understand key values and practise with honesty. Although not all of your team members may be regulated by a professional body, they should all still be following certain employer standards and values. However, many healthcare professionals do have a professional body regulating their role, including the General Medical Council for doctors or the Health and Care Professionals Council, which covers many different professionals, including physiotherapists, dieticians, occupational therapists and many more. Acting as professionals will certainly help a team to work more efficiently; however, individual personalities also contribute to successful teamwork. For example, the Myers-Briggs Personality Type Indicator (MBTI) has been used widely in healthcare practice for many years now to assess a person's preferences and attitudes based on four psychological functions: feeling, thinking, sensation and intuition (Jung, 2014). Understanding what personal attributes each team member will be bringing with them can help the leader to delegate roles and responsibilities appropriately, as well as prevent any future conflict developing. Terry (2020) also highlighted that minimal understanding of personality traits and identities of team members has been perceived as a barrier to effective team working. However, as we discussed above, working towards similar professional values and guidelines helps the team to develop common traits. This is where a positive attitude towards collaborative approach is essential, as you get to know your colleagues but also develop your own emotional intelligence.

Increasing staff satisfaction, morale and well-being

We will begin this section by looking at a case study, which will provide a possible situation you may find yourself in at some point in your training. We will then explore possible solutions towards resolving this situation and steps that can be taken to prevent it in the future.

Case study: Alma

After experiencing some resistance from her colleagues on the acute medical unit about her new role, Alma decided to speak to one of the senior charge nurses – Andy. She expressed her concerns that her colleagues are unsure of her role, sometimes making her feel that she is not contributing to an already very busy workload. Alma also shared that this has caused her a lot of anxiety and she has been feeling anxious coming to work, and more recently, considered stepping away from the TNA course because of it.

Andy understood that the current situation has influenced Alma's well-being and wanted to make sure that any further distress is prevented. He also explained to Alma that her role is very important within the team and that her contribution to patient care is valued by her colleagues, patients and their families. He listened to Alma and suggested contacting Alma's personal tutor at university, who may be able to further support them in tackling this issue.

Andy, Alma and her personal tutor had a meeting to discuss Alma's progress and how she is adapting to her new role as a TNA. Her personal tutor advised that Alma needs to be proactive in communicating effectively with her team, especially in advocating for her new role and her abilities. They further discussed that it would be beneficial for Andy to discuss Alma's new role at the next team meeting. This would provide the team with knowledge on TNA roles and responsibility, and their apprenticeship programme.

Within the next two months, Alma noticed considerable difference in how her team approached her. Following the team meeting, registered nurses were involving Alma in nursing care decision making and made her feel part of the team. She now felt increasingly more confident in using new knowledge gained at university to escalate her concerns and make suggestions to nursing colleagues, doctors and other specialists, such as physiotherapists. Finally feeling part of the team meant that Alma was looking forward to coming to work and felt increasingly satisfied and confident within her developing role.

A feeling of belonging and contributing to shared goals within the unit prevented any further anxiety for Alma. This demonstrates how important teamwork is for increased staff satisfaction and morale. Having good morale within the team helps individuals like Alma to stay motivated to continue developing within their role and give them confidence in communicating effectively with team members about patient care. Job satisfaction can be as important as being competent in specific practical skills. For example, if you did not feel happy and comfortable within your team, you may be reluctant to ask for help when you do feel overwhelmed with your workload. This promotes a toxic working environment, which is unsupportive and can lead to lack of trust between team members. A supportive and encouraging environment should therefore be maintained, where everyone looks out for each other and recognises signs of their team members getting overwhelmed.

Alma was feeling supported by Andy, who represents the management or leader within this team. It also meant that issues were addressed immediately, before escalating further. Andy also sought support from Alma's university tutor, to ensure that he makes informed decisions in this situation. Andy understood that if nothing was done, staff would continue to resist the change in a new addition to the team, thus impacting not only on Alma's well-being but also potentially patient care. If, for example, Alma did not feel confident in speaking to a registered nurse about a change in a patient's observations, it could go unnoticed leading to a risk in patient safety and potential harm. This situation was handled very well by Andy, who recognised the need for staff education, positive staff morale and a reminder of the shared goal. However, not all situations can be or are resolved immediately, leading to barriers in team working and potential conflict.

Activity 3.4   Reflection

Consider a time when you have experienced conflict within a team.

Use SWOT (Strengths, Weaknesses, Opportunities and Threats) analysis to reflect on the situation, particularly focusing on the opportunities that could be taken from the situation (Humphrey, 1970).

Barriers in teams

So far, we have discussed attributes of what makes a good team (Activity 1.2 encouraged you to reflect on your own team's characteristics and possible answers were discussed at the end of this chapter). To develop your understanding further, you need to think about the potential challenges or barriers which prevent teams working effectively to reach their common outcome.

Activity 3.5   Critical thinking

Discuss with your practice assessor or supervisor the below question. They may be able to share their own experiences of working as part of the team or even from the point of leading the team.

Do all teams work well together? Why/why not?

A possible answer outline is given at the end of this chapter. You may find the below discussion useful in formulating your answer.

You may have thought of a variety of challenges, some of which are very specific to your area of work. The challenges that you observed can vary due to the setting of the work environment, organisational dynamics and most importantly service user needs. However, one of the biggest barriers that many teams face is lack of communication among healthcare providers who come from many different settings. While effective communication enables teams to work together to enhance patient care, lack of communication can lead to errors and breakdown in teamwork. Using communication tools, regular team meetings and appropriate policies in place can help to overcome this particular challenge. These tools ensure that each member within a team is up to date with any changes in patient care planning and are able to continue working towards the shared outcome. Improved communication also means that all agencies/disciplines remain vigilant about any changes and provide person-centred care to the individual.

Earlier, we discussed the importance of good leadership within a team. A good leader ensures that good methods of communication are in place within the team and that high standards are maintained, for example, ensuring high quality of handover between team members at all times. This communication method can be very effective, but only if it is implemented appropriately. While a leader gives direction and monitors progress, there needs to be a team on the receiving end of this direction to implement any actions needed and make progress within the set goal. This adds another dimension to an effective team, as we explore the concept of being a follower.

Activity 3.6   Critical thinking

Do you think you can be a leader without having followers?

As this activity is based on your own critical thinking, no outline answer is provided at the end of this chapter.

You may have had an idea in your head that a leader works alone, as they are usually in a senior position within a workplace and lead a team towards a specific goal. However, as Barr and Dowding (2019) highlight, there cannot be leaders without followers as there wouldn't be anybody to lead. This is especially true in healthcare, where teams are often very complex and a leader is relying on individuals to communicate their progress back to the leader, effectively communicate with other team members (followers) and complete their tasks to a good standard. Therefore, you must ensure that while you are still developing your skills of being a good leader, you need to also be a good follower within your team. This may sound complicated and another task for you to do, but what it actually means is being supportive of your colleagues and your leader, demonstrating willingness to learn skills and teach others, and remain professional throughout. This can pose another barrier in teams, if the leader does not have the support of the followers. Problems such as lack of communication, lack of motivation and willingness to learn, difficulty in escalating concerns can soon affect the dynamics of the team and therefore affect patient care.

Developing your professional identity

Case study: Alma

Alma has now been a trainee nursing associate for almost six months. She still regularly finds herself in between the role of healthcare assistance and trainee nursing associate. She is aware that her official title is TNA; however, her team also regularly ask her to carry out tasks of the healthcare assistant, where she is not able to get supervised exposure to new healthcare skills. Although Alma doesn't mind and understands this is part of her role, she cannot help but worry if she is making enough progress in developing within her new role. Alma is feeling unsure about who to speak to about this and is also worried she may appear ungrateful for the opportunity or that she does not want to contribute to a busy team.

Alma's experience in the above case study links to establishment of a professional identity. Haghighat et al. (2020) defined professional identity as a set of values and beliefs that an individual has about their job. This is also shaped by their attitude and moral values, which are further guided by the professional bodies, such as the Nursing and Midwifery Council. Alma has had a clear idea of what her professional identity was; she was a very experienced healthcare assistant, who was confident in her job role within the acute medical unit, had a good relationship with her colleagues, who trusted her to provide best patient care and escalate any concerns she's had. She has a good work ethic, was always punctual and communicated well. However, since becoming a TNA, she was no longer sure what her role was within her team, believing that it should be considerably different straightaway. Feelings of uncertainty, especially when starting a new role, are very valid and should be reflected on. At the same time, further understanding of the process of developing a professional identity would be helpful to Alma, as she would be aware what to expect and what is expected of her.

Before we have a look at what influences development of professional identity, take a look at the below reflective activity. This will help you to consider where you are in your journey to developing your own identity within your current role and how this fits within your team.

Activity 3.7   Reflection

How would you describe your current professional identity? What is important to you when you think about your current role within a team?

If you have just started your journey as a TNA, your current professional identity may still be in development, however you should still be able to discuss your values and morals that you think are important to you within your role.

An outline answer is provided at the end of this chapter.

Table 3.1 Factors influencing professional identity development

What influences professional identity development?	Why is it important?
Role modelling	A positive role model can have a big impact on your development as a healthcare professional. It helps you to identify the qualities that you should be thriving to have and achieve whilst training and beyond. Having a positive role model within Nursing Associate profession can further help you to develop self-confidence and awareness on how you fit in within a team. However, you should be trying to use your own judgment and ensure that your role model has values that uphold the profession. This means following standards set out by the NMC (2018a) and their employer values, as a minimum.
Work Environment and values	Work environment which strives for excellence in patient care, uses evidence-based research to provide care, works as a team and supports continuous professional development, will enable you to secure the feeling of belonging. Every work environment should have a shared goal, to which all team members focused on. The values that work place sets are also very important, as they will influence your own individual values development; especially when you are still new to your role.
Knowledge and skills	The NMC (2018a) state that all TNA's must meet the requirements set out within *Standards of Proficiency*, including Annex A and B. Having particular skills and competencies will help you identify as a competent professional within your field. However, it is important to point out that knowledge and skills alone do not form a professional identity, as many may think. Many factors, including those within this table, contribute to you developing your professional identity. You can be deemed competent in many clinical skills, however without certain values and morals, your professional identity may need further development.
Individual morals and values	Everyone is an individual and you will bring your own morals and values to your profession. These may change throughout your lifetime and also throughout your training to become a qualified NA, as you learn new concepts and get familiar with *The Code* and *Standards of Proficiency for Nursing Associates*.

In the case study, Alma is still at the start of her journey as a TNA and therefore some of the factors which influence her professional identity, such as knowledge, skills and behaviours, are yet to be achieved (Institute of Apprenticeships, 2021). On the other hand, Alma has already got experience working within her work base and is therefore familiar with the work environment and its values. She may already have colleagues who she looks up to, such as registered nurses, doctors or other allied healthcare professionals. Positive role modelling does not have to necessarily come from someone in the same profession as you, but they may possess values and attitudes that you find admirable. As discussed in the table above (2.1), it is important that staff who you work with demonstrate professionalism at all times. Day-Calder (2016) point out that new members of the team often want to fit in within their new team, which unfortunately, may mean they can be easily influenced to change their values. This may refer to good and bad behaviours. This is why finding a positive role model, who adheres to high professional and patient care standards, will enable new staff, like Alma, to continue developing their professional identity.

Thinking that professional identity is developed at the beginning of your career as a TNA/NA can create a barrier in your development. Continuous professional development (CPD) is part of all healthcare professionals' responsibilities, as they progress in their careers, learn new skills and gain new knowledge. It has also recently become part of nursing and nursing associate guidelines, set out by the NMC, as we are required to revalidate every few years, to demonstrate continuous learning and commitment to excellent quality of patient care. CPD means that as you gain new knowledge and experience, as well as disregard values and certain experiences, your professional identity will also change alongside it (Slusser et al., 2018). This is a process that you will engage in throughout your career and which will be highly influenced by colleagues, educators and your work environment (Slusser et al., 2018). You will learn more about CPD and the importance of keeping up to date with latest practice, later in this book.

Alma's lack of confidence could also be linked to her lack of understanding of other healthcare professionals' roles and how her new role fits in, especially on her ward. NMC (2018a) outlines what Alma's responsibility is, within *Standards of Proficiency for Nursing Associates*:

4.1. Demonstrate an awareness of the roles, responsibilities and scope of practice of different members of the nursing and interdisciplinary team, and their own role within it.

Understanding the 'scope of practice' of members within a team would allow Alma to be more confident in what her role is and when she should seek support or input from others, when it comes to patient care needs. Campbell (2020) further adds that members within a team need to be aware of their own strengths and weaknesses, which would allow recognition of own practice limitations and therefore lead to escalation/referral of care. Alma therefore has the responsibility to find out what professionals her work base team is made up of. For Alma, who works within the adult acute medical unit, obvious professionals may include: nurses, doctors (including specialist doctors), healthcare assistants, radiographers and other acute care specialists. However, as Alma develops within her role and gets exposed to other fields of healthcare practice, she will need to be aware of other professions. For example, for her next practice exposure/placement, Alma may be placed within a paediatric mental health setting and will need to be aware of professionals, such as dietitians, psychologists, art therapists, music therapists and learning disability link nurses.

Activity 3.8   Research

See below some of the examples of allied health professions. Take a minute to think about each of them and if you know what their role is. If unsure, research and find out more about what they do (This list is not exhaustive and many more professions could be added, depending on the healthcare setting discussed).

Art therapists
Drama therapists
Chiropodists
Occupational therapists
Operating department practitioners
Radiographers
Speech and language therapists
Prosthetists and orthotists
Dieticians
*List derived from NHS England – The 14 allied health professions
As this activity is based on your own research, no outline answer is provided at the end of this chapter.

Chapter summary

Interdisciplinary team working is an essential part of providing excellent care in practice. However, it comes with many challenges, due to barriers in communication, personality types, leadership issues and many more that have been discussed within this chapter. Integrating the role of a nursing associate within interdisciplinary teams can therefore be very challenging, but far from impossible. The nursing associate role has been created to bridge the gap in care, allowing NAs to fit within existing teams. NMC (2018a) provide clear guidelines within Platform 4 of *Standard of Proficiencies for Nursing Associates*, focusing on 'Working in Teams'. Training for NAs is therefore based on this platform, to ensure that once you qualify, you are able to recognise your own role within teams and use your critical thinking skills to identify when there are issues in teams working well together.

Activities: Brief outline answers

Activity 3.1 Reflective and critical thinking (page 44)

1. Some of the key elements of teamwork you have considered may include:

   - good communication skills (with colleagues and patients);
   - everyone understanding their own job roles, as well as each other's;
   - mutual priorities established;
   - good leadership;
   - continuous professional development individually and as a team;
   - ability to speak up and raise concerns in a safe manner;
   - democratic approach.

   (Adapted from Reeves et al., 2010)

2. You may find that to complete the first activity, you used your team as an example of identifying important team characteristics. This is absolutely fine, however, consider how other teams may differ. If your work base, for example, is within adult learning disability services, consider what different skills and attributes teams may need to have within children's field of nursing? This may include more emphasis on a family-centred care approach and many more professionals involved in a team, which would not be the same for your field of nursing.

3. Your team may not be good at meeting some of the attributes above and this could be due to a variety of reasons. These may include organisational issues, performance management issues, and inappropriate skill mix or could be due to individual personalities within the team.

Activity 3.2 Scenario assessment (page 46)

1. Patients may experience a variety of emotional and cognitive changes following a stroke. In this scenario, there is an added aspect of Jonathan being a young adult, who has now had to put his life plans completely on hold and focus on his recovery.

He would be possibly feeling that he is not in control of his body and his life, perhaps comparing himself to his friends who were now at university doing what he wanted to do. This can have a huge impact on his mental health and therefore his motivation towards recovery and rehabilitation. It is very important to consider all aspects of a patient's recovery using a holistic approach, rather than just focusing on their physical needs. The person-centred approach to care within a team will be further discussed later in the book.

2. You may have thought of involving someone from the mental health team, such as a psychiatrist or a therapist. This would help with Jonathan's emotional rehabilitation following a stroke and help him to come up with coping strategies, while undergoing the challenging rehabilitation process.

Activity 3.5 Critical thinking (page 50)

Hopefully, you have been able to have a discussion with your practice assessor/supervisor about teamwork in general. You may have discussed that some teams work very well together, as they share the same values and goals, have perhaps worked together for a while and complement one another's personalities. However, you have most likely had a conversation about teams not always working together effectively. There may be many reasons for this, including the barriers that we have discussed within the chapter. Individual personalities, work culture and values can affect the team, who may find it difficult to maintain effective working relationships. We discuss tools for teamwork later in this book.

Activity 3.7 Reflection (page 52)

Within your reflection you may have included certain values such as: honesty, reliability, determination, accountability and highlighted some important skills such as listening, being a good communicator and ensuring you are competent within your role. These sets of values, together with a feeling of belonging within a team, lead to development of your professional identity. There is no right answer when it comes to how you feel within your role, as everyone will have slightly different values. This is also why it is important that healthcare professions, such as nursing associates, have professional guidelines to follow as well as their own personal values. This ensures that there is a minimum standard for professional identity; the rest comes from you and your experience.

Further reading

Health Education England (HEE) (2021) *Working Differently Together: Progressing a One Workforce Approach.* www.hee.nhs.uk/sites/default/files/documents/HEE_MDT_Toolkit_V1.1.pdf

Toolkit developed by HEE in partnership with NHS, supporting development of interdisciplinary teams in healthcare. Includes some very useful resources within referencing and bibliography.

Useful websites

www.hee.nhs.uk/our-work/nursing-associates

Health Education England (HEE) page for nursing associates. An essential resource for background around NA role development and resources evaluating integration of the role into healthcare practices.

www.nice.org.uk/guidance/ng128

National Institute for Health and Care Excellence (NICE) (2022) *Stroke and Transient Ischaemic Attack in Over 16s: Diagnosis and Initial Management.*

To develop further knowledge on management of stroke, search the link above. Keeping up to date with the latest guidelines is your responsibility as a learner and once you become a qualified nursing associate.

www.belbin.com/about/belbin-team-roles

Belbin teamwork theory. Details around steps within Belbin teamwork theory are covered within this page. There are many different team working theories out there and they are chosen appropriately for team requirements.

https://assets.publishing.service.gov.uk/government/uploads/system/uploads/attachment_data/file/279124/0947.pdf

Francis, R (2013) *Report of the Mid Staffordshire NHS Foundation Trust Public Inquiry. Executive Summary.*

This is another essential read. Nursing associate role development was hugely associated with this report and informed future practice, and requirement for change.

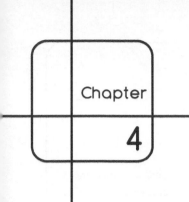

Chapter

4

How to deliver and contribute to person-centred care within a team

NMC STANDARDS OF PROFICIENCY FOR NURSING ASSOCIATES

This chapter will address the following platforms and proficiencies:

Platform 3: Provide and monitor care

At the point of registration, the registered nursing associate will be able to:

3.4   demonstrate the knowledge, communication and relationship management skills required to provide people, families and carers with accurate information that meets their needs before, during and after a range of interventions

3.5   work in partnership with people, to encourage shared decision making, in order to support individuals, their families and carers to manage their own care when appropriate

3.18   demonstrate the ability to monitor the effectiveness of care in partnership with people, families and carers. Document progress and report outcomes

Platform 4: Working in teams

At the point of registration, the registered nursing associate will be able to:

4.1   demonstrate an awareness of the roles, responsibilities, and scope of practice of different members of the nursing and interdisciplinary team, and their role within it

4.2   demonstrate an ability to support and motivate other members of the care team and interact confidently with them

Platform 6: Contributing to integrated care

At the point of registration, the registered nursing associate will be able to:

6.1   understand the roles of the different providers of health and care. Demonstrate the ability to work collaboratively and in partnership with professionals from different agencies in interdisciplinary teams

6.4   understand the principles and processes involved in supporting people and families with a range of care needs to maintain optimal independence and avoid unnecessary interventions and disruptions to their lives

Introduction

Person-centred care (PCC) as a concept has been widely used within healthcare as a means of understanding the perceived needs of an individual and incorporating those needs in the care you provide. If you were asked what person-centred care means to you, you may also state that it is an approach that facilitates a therapeutic relationship between patient and healthcare professional. You would be correct in thinking so, however, this chapter will prompt you to explore the basics of person-centred care to fundamentally understand what it is to be person-centred working in healthcare today within a team. People want to be treated with dignity and respect; this means not to be merely seen as a body part or problem. Through the chapter you will be guided to think of the person first and then the disease, ensuring you are able to identify the wider influences that impact on how healthcare delivery is organised, managed and delivered to ensure people as individuals, communities and populations are at the heart of planning and policy making.

Person-centred care is a broad subject and for you as a nursing associate, you are in a unique position to be working with individuals and their families from all four fields of nursing. This brings its own challenges to consider as you will need to understand the needs of all of these four fields to truly achieve person-centred outcomes for the communities you serve. The chapter will allow you to explore all four fields of nursing through specific case study scenarios relevant to each specific field of nursing. Irrespective of which care environment you work in as a nursing associate, the NMC requires patients to be treated with respect. You will have the opportunity to apply learning from Chapter 1 to explore how the attitudes and behaviours of a nursing associate inform and support the culture and practices within the environment you work in. This will be achieved through focusing on fostering partnership and communication within teams through team working.

Understanding person-centredness

Patient-centred care has been an evolving concept, originally a term characterised by Enid Balint in 1969 as understanding the patient as a 'unique' being, to more recently with the widely used 'Person-Centred Nursing Framework' developed by McCormack and McCance in 2006. They describe PCC as *an approach to practice, established through formation and fostering of healthful relationships between all care providers ... underpinned by values of respect for persons* (McCormack and McCance, 2017). The philosophy underpinning the framework embeds the concept depicted by Enid Balint which explores the concept of being a 'person', focusing on what it means to be human. You may question how this philosophical approach relates to the delivery of PCC in your practice. The following activity has been designed so you are able to reflect on what it means to you to be seen as a 'person'.

Activity 4.1   Reflection

We suggest writing your thoughts down, so you can refer back to your notes.

Make a list of the attributes and characteristics you deem to be important to be seen as a 'person'. You may consider physical and psychological characteristics that define a person, yet you may also explore this further to include components such as the importance of your feelings, emotions and desires.

Now reflect on the following questions:

- Do you think if a person loses any of the attributes and characteristics you have listed through disease and disability, they are seen as less of a person?
- What about caring for someone who has had a leg amputated due to disease or the woman who has had a double mastectomy due to a cancer diagnosis?
- A new mother who has refused to see her newborn baby but is diagnosed with psychosis?

As this activity is based on your own thoughts, no outline answer is provided at the end of this chapter.

Your reflections on this activity will differ widely with other nursing associates. This shows every individual is unique in their own understanding of what it means to be seen as a person. The complexities of this means every individual will have different thoughts to you in regard to this, but you will likely all agree that it is a fundamental human need to be recognised as a person. This activity also highlights the necessity of self-awareness through self-reflection. Person-centred practice requires personal insight into one's own and others' values. In Chapter 1 you had the opportunity to reflect on your personal and professional values that have an impact on your responses when you directly provide care to patients and families. These values and attitudes of the individual and team are key in achieving person-centred approaches in care planning and delivery.

Principles of PCC

In 2019 the NHS Long Term Plan set out a ten-year strategic plan which described five major changes to the NHS service model, one of which is:

People will get more control over their own health, and more personalised care when they need it.

The personalised care strategy that was proposed sets out key skills, knowledge and activities that the workforce will need to provide so that person-centred care can be delivered in a personalised way. The relevance of the strategy is closely applicable to your understanding of how integrated care across sectors such as health, social care, local authorities, housing and private sectors relies on teamwork to deliver a seamless plan of care.

To be able to gain a further understanding into how policy shapes the way you practise as a nursing associate, read the following boxes that will provide an overview of each document.

Understanding the theory: the key documents

Five Year Forward View (2014)

This document sets a clear direction of where the NHS wants to be. It focuses on four key chapters from why the NHS needs to change, to what the future will look like, most notably for you as a nursing associate. Chapter 2 focuses on the relationship with patients and communities. For you to be able to implement this into your practice the document explores themes of empowerment and engagement of communities that you work with. As a nursing associate you can positively contribute to this. Your scope of practice incorporates promoting the health and well-being of patients in the communities they live in. The document allows you to explore how this can be achieved in a person-centred way, allowing patients to increase the direct control they have over the care that is provided to them through increased choice over where and how they receive care. Secondly, there is an emphasis on an integrated approach with stronger partnership working with voluntary organisations to work alongside the NHS.

The Five Year Forward View for Mental Health (2016)

This key document sets out priority changes for the transformation of NHS mental health services in England by the year 2021. Key priorities included a seven-day NHS with increased access to early intervention services for mental health conditions such as psychosis. An important aspect of the strategy was the need for an integrated mental and physical health approach. This means as a nursing associate you would need to be aware that the strategy encouraged the need for both physical and mental health to be seen equally as important. This requires an understanding of a person-centred approach when providing care to patients. Children and young people's mental health services is where the strategy has set the most ambitious plans whereby funding will grow faster than both overall NHS funding and total mental health spending. Since its inception, the NHS mental health implementation plan 2019/20–2023/24 will now provide a new framework to ensure commitments are delivered.

The Care Act (2014)

This Act represents the most significant reform of care and support in more than 60 years, putting people and their carers in control of their care and support. As a nursing associate you need to have an understanding as to how the Care Act intends to do this. One of the main overarching principles of the Act is the patient knows best, patients are 'experts by experience' who need to be encouraged to think about what outcomes they want to achieve in their lives enabling a greater sense of physical or emotional well-being. While as a nursing associate you will not be undertaking assessment of needs independently, and will be supervised by a registered nurse, the foremost message from the Act sets out clear criteria as to how assessments need to change to include involvement of the patient/service user.

The theory box above provides an overview of three important documents that have led to the need for an approach that puts people at the centre of their care. The personalised care strategy sets out the model *The Comprehensive Model of Personalised Care* (NHS England, 2018), which defines the following six core activities that happen across health and social care services:

- shared decision making;
- personalised care & support planning;

- self-management support;
- social prescribing and community-based approaches;
- personalised budgets;
- enabling choice.

The purpose of these core activities is so that as many people as possible can benefit throughout their lives through an integrated approach of personalised care. This integrated approach requires teamwork at its core, which will be discussed later in this chapter. To apply this to your current practice, you will be asked to consider the following knowledge and activities advocated by the model and explore how as a nursing associate you apply them in practice.

- *The core of person-centred approaches:* these include values, your own attitudes, behaviours, communication and relationship-building skills, conversations to engage with people, conversations to enable and support people
- *Knowledge:* social determinants of health, quality improvement, co-production, health literacy, patient activation
- *Activities:* shared decision making, care co-ordination, care and support planning, care navigation, supporting self-management, making every contact count, working in partnership at individual and service level, advanced care planning

(HEE, 2020)

Teamwork

One of the core activities of the model is shared decision making. In healthcare today organisations consist of culturally diverse and skilled interdisciplinary team members. While each speciality will have a specific focus in that patient's care, the unified goal for all is to provide a positive patient experience, which essentially requires teamwork. There are multiple definitions of what teams and teamwork is described to be discussed in Chapter 3. Fundamentally the word 'team' can be defined as two or more individuals who work co-operatively through a framework to successfully complete a task (D'Angelo, 2019). While this may seem like a basic definition, the accomplishment of the goal is through collaboration between two or more individuals. This collaboration will also include patients and their families who are contributing members of the team. To understand each key individual who is part of the team it is imperative team members are knowledgeable about one another's roles and responsibilities, providing a framework in which each team member's skills are best recognised in the patient's plan of care. So as a nursing associate you need to consider which essential skills, knowledge and behaviours you bring that contribute towards your role within a team. The following activity will allow you to explore the specific knowledge, skills and behaviours that are aligned to the profession.

Activity 4.2   Critical thinking

Access the *Standards of Proficiency for Nursing Associates* (NMC, 2018a) and refer to ' Annex A' and 'Annex B' (pages 18-26). You are required to make a list of the necessary knowledge, skills and behaviours that you think are required to work in teams collaborating effectively with a range of health and social care professionals. Annexes A and B cover a broad range of clinical and communication skills; you are only required to identify the skills and procedures directly related to team working.

(Continued)

(Continued)

As part of your critical thinking, consider the following questions:

- Who are the key people who you will engage to achieve this?
- What are your strengths and areas of development to achieve this?
- Why is this skill relevant in your role as a nursing associate?

An outline answer is provided at the end of the chapter.

Your professional standards explicitly describe the essential nature of communication (essential skill) in managing relationships with people (these include both patients, families and members of the team) in the provision of high-quality person-centred care. You may have identified active listening as an essential interpersonal skill within team working, but how does this skill impact on patient care directly? The *Report of the Mid Staffordshire NHS Foundation Trust Public Inquiry* (The Francis Report, 2013) highlighted many failings in aspects of care considered so central to nursing that these fundamentals of care central to patient safety were overlooked. Out of the 290 recommendations made by the Francis Report (2013) there was a strong emphasis on improving support for compassionate, caring and committed nursing. What does this mean to patients you care for? You may argue these are core values that you already demonstrate in practice, but how do you demonstrate these in practice? To be able to provide care that is caring and compassionate, you need to demonstrate a basic ability to communicate effectively with the patients you care for in teams you work in. Hargie and Dickson (2004) propose a model of communication called *A Skill Model of Interpersonal Communication*. This model of communication is particularly relevant to the application of person-centred care as it recognises successful communication as being focused and purposeful. The context in which individuals communicate has been identified by being underpinned by the following six elements:

1. person-centred context
2. goals
3. mediating processes
4. responses
5. feedback
6. perception

(Hargie and Dickson, 2004)

As an overview these six elements are imperative when working within a team where the goal is to deliver safe, effective care in a collaborative manner. You also need to consider the effects of your own actions within this communication process (mediating processes) to then be able to modify your actions (responses and feedback from others) in light of the information shared by others. In teams this is encouraged through team reflection activities and with patients and service users this is encouraged through feedback. While I have provided a brief overview of the elements, I want to bring to your attention the importance of reflection in the communication process.

To better understand the key elements of the model and its application through shared decision making being a key principle of PCC you are encouraged to read the case study and complete the activities related to it.

Case study: Mohammed

Mohammed, a nursing associate, works within the school nurse team; his primary role is to support the school nurse with undertaking health assessments of youths entering the youth offending system. He is new to his role as he has recently qualified as a nursing associate. While he previously worked with children and young people in an acute setting, this speciality is not familiar. He is keen to learn and is very motivated.

During their weekly assessment clinic at the local youth offending centre, they meet 15-year-old Tyler who has attended for his health assessment. Tyler has a history of anti-social behaviour and has recently been referred to the team by the police to be enrolled on to the youth crime prevention programme.

The school nurse takes the lead in undertaking the assessment while Mohammed contributes to it. Tyler is very reluctant to communicate and shares that he doesn't want to be here, and he will not talk. Mohammed asks why this is and Tyler responds by saying he doesn't trust anyone and 'you are all the same'. Mohammed continues to ask questions and the school nurse states that if Tyler does not want to talk then his wishes should be respected. After a brief silence Tyler speaks. They are able to gather information about Tyler's health: he has been diagnosed with asthma, is a regular smoker and he cannot remember attending the GP surgery to review his asthma. He has medication prescribed for his asthma. He occasionally smokes cannabis and shares that nobody else is aware of this. Tyler has been excluded from mainstream school and is attending alternative education. Mohammed asks about his family relationships and if he has a support network around him. Tyler states that he does not have a good relationship with his mother and his father doesn't live with them. He has many good friends, and he trusts them.

In the above case study, Mohammed needs to identify which healthcare professionals and agencies are involved as part of the collaborative process that will contribute to Tyler's care plan. The care plan will ultimately inform Mohammed about the roles of those in the interdisciplinary team and how they contribute towards shared treatment goals.

Activity 4.3   Research

Make a list or draw a diagram of those who you think should be involved in contributing towards Tyler's plan of care.

Critically evaluate the following person-centred questions to inform your list/diagram.

- What are Tyler's needs? Think about Tyler holistically and not just his physical needs.
- Who is best at addressing those needs? While the school nurse may support Tyler with advice around smoking cessation, is she the best person to provide long-term support in regard to this?
- What are the goals of each intervention?
- What skills are required by Mohammed to contribute to this assessment?

An outline answer is provided at the end of the chapter.

By completing this activity you would have been able to identify the importance of an integrated team approach to care delivery (this will be discussed further in the chapter). Integration of care is a key dimension of PCC. If you refer to the six elements of the model advocated by Hargie and Dickson (2004) and the *The Comprehensive Model of Personalised Care* which has been mentioned earlier in the chapter, you will be able to identify the relevance of the two models. Hargie and Dickson (2004) advocate communication needs to be undertaken in a person-centred context; this means individuals will bring with them their own personal values, expectations and dispositions to an encounter (as witnessed by Tyler) which will have an impact on the outcome of the assessment if the patient/service user needs are not understood or listened to. Working together in mutual partnership with Tyler through the assessment process will also allow the key activities stated in the *The Comprehensive Model of Personalised Care* (NHS, 2018) of shared decision making, co-ordinating care and working in partnership at individual level to be successfully implemented.

The nursing process and team working

The nursing process has five stages according to Howatson-Jones et al. (2005). These processes were adapted by Harris (2021) for nursing associates. As a nursing associate you will be contributing to and delivering patient care prescribed by the plan of care for an individual. You will be taking a systematic approach to managing your patients' needs through this evidence-based approach. The process can be used as a guide across all four fields of nursing in any speciality which you may be exposed to. The recognition and participation of the interdisciplinary team is integral in the nursing process as they will essentially form the prescribed plan of care for the patient. Although as a nursing associate you will not write a care plan, it is within your scope of practice to be able to evaluate them. You will most likely work alongside the registered nurse to suggest changes and make updates to them. It is a communication tool between members of the multidisciplinary team and will also consider the roles of the wider interdisciplinary team and their roles. You can now critically reflect on applying the nursing process and explore how members of the wider team contribute to the patient's plan of care. You have already established key members who should be involved in Tyler's plan of care; you will now explore this in relation to the nursing process.

Activity 4.4   Critical thinking

The five stages of the nursing process are stated below. You need to complete each stage by providing a brief definition of each; this will provide some context to what your understanding of each stage is. You are then asked to consider which members of the interdisciplinary and multidisciplinary teams are involved at each stage. You will need to provide a rationale as to why they may need to be involved in contributing to Tyler's plan of care. To provide you with some guidance we have completed the first stage for you.

- **Assessment** – Is the first step which forms the foundation of ascertaining the patient's/ service user's health status. At this stage you will use a patient assessment tool to collect information about the patient's needs. Each field of nursing will have specific assessment tools that will be used in practice while others may use generic assessment tools. The aim is to identify signs of deterioration, or any red flags displayed by the patient. This process will include collecting of objective and subjective data related to the physical, psychological, social, developmental, cultural and spiritual status of the patient/service user.

In relation to Tyler's case study, all team members who are present during the assessment process will contribute to assessing the patient. Mohammed and the registered nurse will share feedback from their observations and the information they have collected. This provides increased accountability to all team members present rather than just one member of the team who is in a senior position. As a nursing associate you have a duty to contribute to ongoing assessment of the patient but the overall responsibility of formulating a plan of care will be the registered nurse's responsibility. Therefore, clear communication is paramount for effective partnership working. Tyler is the other individual who is integral to the assessment process as he will identify his needs during the process and the process will be guided by him.

- **Patient goals**
- **Planning**
- **Implementation**
- **Evaluation**

A brief outline to this activity is provided at the end of the chapter.

While you were undertaking this activity you may have identified the key underlying principle of developing a therapeutic relationship with Tyler, enabling him to feel comfortable to speak about his feelings. This then allows the school nurse and Mohammed to explore and address his concerns. Essentially the nursing associate, nurse and patient/service user share both power and responsibility relating to the care planned. At this point as a nursing associate, you will negotiate which needs of the care plan will need to be shared with other care team members with Tyler exercising his power of informed consent to progress this. Price (2019) states patients will choose and specify how they prefer to collaborate with healthcare professionals. The patient then becomes an expert on their illness. Partnership in care involves the negotiation of expectations and responsibilities. As a nursing associate you also need to recognise that some expectations may be unrealistic. How do you navigate around those challenges but also maintain patient autonomy? As a nursing associate you will need to navigate around these complexities by having knowledge about the possible challenges that face each different field of nursing. If we consider Activity 4.4, Tyler is an adolescent, so how much choice can he be given in terms of treatment and care? What is Tyler's role in the collaborative process? Does he have the capabilities to participate? These questions are imperative as Tyler is a key member of the 'team' and these questions will essentially determine his role and responsibility in PCC.

Activity 4.5   Reflection and person-centred care approaches

Consider the following four fields of nursing and reflect on the possible complexities which need to be considered in relation to shared decision making when working with patients/service users from these fields. Also, think about the wider team and their role in this process. You may find this activity is best undertaken by speaking to other trainee nursing associates who work in other fields different to you.

- children;
- adults;

(Continued)

(Continued)

- learning disabilities;
- mental health.

As this activity is based on your own thoughts, no outline answer is provided at the end of this chapter.

During this activity you would have found that shared decision making starts with the conversation between the person receiving care and the person/people delivering care. It puts people at the centre of decisions about their own treatment and care. However, the activity would have also highlighted the possible conflict between professional judgement and expertise and balancing this with the needs and wishes of the person receiving care. You may have also explored the potential conflicts with the decision-making process between health and social care professionals in choosing the right plan of care for the person receiving care. Enabling patients to be active participants in their health and healthcare is a critical goal for the NHS in England. The benefits of this allows the person receiving care to feel supported and empowered to make informed choices, while allowing healthcare professionals to advocate for their patients if possible conflicts do arise between the MDT when deciding on the plan of care for the person.

While the below is not an activity, here are some questions that you may want to consider when you next provide care to patients that you meet:

- How am I working in equal partnership with people who use services and their carers in my role, sharing choice, control and decisions together?
- How do I communicate to others the impact of being person-centred in how we work with people in context of their communities both within populations we serve and the people and staff who work with us?

Interdisciplinary working and PCC

Interdisciplinary teams are an approach to healthcare that integrates multiple disciplines through collaboration. The aim of this collaboration is for patients to receive care that is patient focused through effective communication and teamwork. Multidisciplinary teams differ to interdisciplinary teams in that they work in parallel rather than in integration, each within their respective disciplines to devise their own care plans. For instance, a patient who sustains a leg amputation may receive treatment from an orthopaedic surgeon, occupational therapist, prosthetist, physiotherapist to name a few. Each discipline will have their own goals for the patient and may not consult with one another to discuss treatment. As discussed earlier, when services do not collaboratively work together, this leads to a negative impact on patient outcomes. Integrated care relies on teamwork. With an ageing population and an increase in long-term health conditions it is paramount that services are organised so that they not only minimise costs of preventable illnesses dependency but also reduce inappropriate admissions and prescribed medications. People living with learning disabilities, dementia, multiple long-term conditions, mental and physical conditions together and end-of-life care patients are likely to need care from a range of services (statutory and community) and professionals. Providing a truly person-centred approach means the co-ordination of these services rather than the patient or family members pursuing different services to co-ordinate that care. A useful document that may help your understanding of the importance of PCC and collaboration further, is available through the National Voices web page (www.nationalvoices.org.uk), a coalition of charities that stand for people in control of their health and care. A report undertaken by National Voices (2017) found even though integration is a necessity, patients want co-ordination of care. This means professionals working together as a team around them. Now consider the activity and the case study below.

Activity 4.6   Critical thinking

Interdisciplinary working not only benefits patients but healthcare professionals alike. Read the case study below and then answer the following questions.

- What are the benefits of applying a collaborative approach to patient care?
- What elements are required to achieve a successful interdisciplinary team to provide personalised care?

As this is based on your own reflection, an outline answer is not provided at the end of this chapter.

Case study: Mary

Mary is a 67-year-old retired nurse. She was diagnosed with type 2 diabetes 15 years ago. She has raised cholesterol and had a stroke three years ago. She also is under the Congenital Heart Condition team at the local hospital. The community nurses visit her daily to monitor her diabetes. She also has osteoporosis which affects her mobility. She has been living on her own since the death of her husband five years ago. Her daughter visits her once a week to help with any household chores. Mary is becoming increasingly forgetful and at times gets confused with where she is.

While answering the questions did you think of the following:

- **Improved care and outcomes**

Healthcare professionals in separate disciplines can provide insights into her condition. In Mary's case these include: the endocrinologist for her osteoporosis, the community nurses monitoring her diabetes, the cardiologist for her heart condition. Each will notice specific symptoms related to their speciality. Individually they can treat one aspect of her condition. However, they can provide comprehensive treatment that addresses her multifaceted symptoms, improving the possibility of a co-ordinated personalised care plan. This, however, requires excellent communication and negotiation skills between services to respond, which means a culture change in how services are arranged.

- **Reduced errors**

Errors such as misdiagnosis, overlooked symptoms and numerous medication prescriptions can be fatal for a patient and can have long-lasting complications. This can be a result of patients seeing numerous services that may not consider prescriptions and diagnosis by another service. A holistic approach to assessing a patient's symptoms means in Mary's care planning, the community nurses can review her current medication in partnership with the endocrinologist and the cardiology team. In successful teams, each member acknowledges and respects the abilities of the other. This involves having an understanding of the extent of their knowledge and areas of overlap with others' disciplines and the knowledge they can learn. For example, the community nurse and GP are both likely to be knowledgeable about Mary's physiological symptoms and any deterioration in her diabetes. Though the GP may be more specialised, they can trust the community nurses to know and treat symptoms.

- **Treatment goals**

The approach encourages awareness of individual needs within the team and encourages communication so that other members have the information they need to apply another aspect of treatment. This improves efficiency and reduces errors and streamlines services. Instead of health professionals giving instructions and advice about what each service will do, the patient is encouraged to identify the support they need to achieve their treatment goals. In Mary's care it is important to involve her daughter in the decision-making process. This can help also support her daughter to identify and seek support and in resources in the community if she so wishes.

- **Shared leadership**

You may be thinking with all the different services involved about how care is managed and co-ordinated. In the interdisciplinary approach, the role of the leader can be fluid. Often, the individual with the most experience and knowledge will be leading others in management. However, the leadership position may shift as the team goes from treating one symptom to another. So, if we look at Mary, her care may first be managed by cardiology due to her congenital heart condition. As her diabetes have been poorly managed this care may have been shifted to the GP and then the community nurses to monitor. With Mary's developing symptoms of confusion, the lead in her care may be transferred back to the GP.

Team-based reflection

For you to deliver and contribute to PCC within a team it is paramount that you take time out to think about what you are doing and why you are doing things that have an impact on other people. When I refer to other people, I am going to focus on other healthcare professionals and professionals from other sectors you work alongside. Self-awareness and participation in reflective practice are recognised as vital to supporting the person-centred care agenda.

Arguably leadership is essential for the implementation of PCC in practice. The NMC (2018b) states that throughout their career, registrants will have opportunities to demonstrate their leadership qualities. For you as a nursing associate, one area of practice you will demonstrate leadership skills will be through service development and quality improvement. What is your role within this to enhance the experiences of care and well-being of patients? This will firstly start with an understanding of the skill needs of the teams you work within. Being able to have this understanding requires self-awareness. Advocators of PCC, McCormack and McCance (2006) who developed the person-centred nursing framework as a tool to enable nurses to explore person-centred care in their practice discuss 'prerequisites'. These 'prerequisites' focus on the attributes of the nurse and stress the importance of nursing staff 'knowing self'. They refer to the nurse, however, it is a concept that can be adopted by all healthcare workers. As a nursing associate how can you work effectively amongst others to deliver the outcomes of care? Simply contributing to care planning does not necessarily mean improved care outcomes. A variety of factors are considered in quality improvement (QI) interventions in clinical settings that have a direct impact on safe, timely, effective and efficient patient-centred care. Quality improvement can be described as giving those involved in delivering care the time and resources to problem solve and bring about improvement through a co-ordinated and systematic approach.

One intervention that is key in healthcare practice and which healthcare staff undertake formally and informally is the practice of reflection. Reflection is mostly an activity individuals identify for professional development, and which is mostly undertaken as an individual activity. Team-based reflective practice is something that is not common practice in the clinical environment. When caring for patients a team approach is utilised and all team members are active key participants in implementing patient care, then why is team reflective practice not commonly used? One such barrier to this may be the perceived lack of time; however, healthcare staff are experiencing unprecedented levels of stress and ill health as a result of not investing time in understanding their own needs (emotional, physical and spiritual) and how these impact on the care they provide to patients in teams they work within. Spurling (2004) refers to the concept of containment whereby an individual shares their state of mind with others so it can be interpreted into something that is tolerable and meaningful. You may ask how does this impact on QI? Meaningful quality improvement goes beyond individual changes; collaboration is required to integrate team-based reflection into interventions which may provide opportunities to facilitate change processes. Team-based reflective practice helps teams in the actual work of problem solving but this will only be effective if there is a recognition of creating a workplace that is conducive to improvement and this involves allowing staff to reflect.

Activity 4.7   Reflection

Think about how team-based reflection within your practice can lead to learning and change (QI).

Provide an example so you are able to reflect on how this quality issue can be problem solved through team-based reflective practice.

As this activity is based on your own reflection, no outline answer is provided at the end of this chapter.

During this activity you may have identified a specific issue within your practice that can lead to change if staff have the capacity to share their experiences. This is the first component of QI, where the quality problem is identified and understood. One example of such an issue can be staff discontent with workload. Recognising why and how that problem has arisen will allow for designing improvement. Teamwork-based reflective practice can allow the process of containment in a safe environment. Everyone in the group reflection will fulfil the role of the 'container'. This will increase the capacity of the individual to share and contain their experience of difficult feelings, allowing others who also have felt overwhelmed with workload to talk about their experiences. What do you think the danger is if these feelings/experiences are not shared with others? Individuals will repeat their actions of feeling discontent leading to a continuous cycle of discontent. Team-based reflection can provide a basis for problem solving and consequently leading to problem-solving actions that involve a team approach.

Chapter summary

This chapter has provided you with an insight into the meaning of providing person-centred care in collaboration with the interdisciplinary team. Recognising the role others play in achieving the care plan goals for a patient requires you as a nursing associate to know what your scope of practice allows you to contribute to care planning. While each profession will have their own specific role within achieving identified goals, you would have established through this chapter the role the patient/service user plays in shared decision making. The tools within the chapter have been created to allow you to consolidate your understanding of the key skills required for collaborative team working, an essential approach that will put people at the centre of their care. Key documents have been explored which will support you in providing a background to the necessity of person-centred care in healthcare. Remember to keep yourself up to date with these documents and others that shape how care is delivered.

Activities: Brief outline answers

Activity 4.2 Critical thinking (page 63)

The ability to communicate effectively, with sensitivity and compassion is central to the provision of person-centred care. Some of the skills you may have explored when referring to skills in Annexes A and B is having the ability to provide clear verbal and written instructions (1.11) when sharing information: this is imperative when working within teams as delegating and handing over responsibility for care to others is a key function in collaborative working. The relevance of communication skills in teams allows for appropriate escalation of concerns (4.2) for a timely response between services. You may have considered a variety of communication skills that contribute to achieving this in a team. Do you employ active listening skills when receiving feedback from team members?

You may have also considered the skills in Annex B which require the ability to apply the communication and management skills to deliver care across the lifespan. An example of this may be utilising support from others to convey messages of compassion and sensitivity (2.9) to meet the care priorities of a dying person and their family or carers (9.2).

Activity 4.3 Research (page 65)

You may have considered the following services/agencies who would be involved in Tyler's care:

- police;
- probation officers;
- social worker;
- school;
- charities;
- drug misuse services;
- smoking cessation;
- asthma nurse;
- GP;
- school nurse.

You may have identified Tyler's emotional health needs; there are relationship struggles with his family and he does not feel he can talk to them. While Tyler does identify as having a friendship support system, this needs to be explored further to establish if this is supportive. There may be a variety of complex reasons why someone may not want to talk about their difficulties. There is a danger that if someone is reluctant to talk, you may not ascertain the core reason that needs to be tackled to provide or support, or a young person may not want to engage at all. The key here is to develop a therapeutic relationship with Tyler. You may explore who may be best placed to provide continuous support. The school nurse will essentially need to liaise with support services for emotional health support, but this will need to be with Tyler's consent. Consent can be obtained, and a needs assessment can only be undertaken when there is trust. This is a basis for any care plan to be implemented where shared decision making is the goal. The asthma nurse will need to be contacted if Tyler has not been reviewed. The school nurse will co-ordinate this care plan. Substance misuse services may be involved through youth offending services to support Tyler with his cannabis use. The school nurse may continue to work with Tyler in regard to his emotional health and refer if long-term support is required.

For Mohammed to involve Tyler in the shared decision making, Mohammed will need to develop his communication and listening skills. His communication skills, both written and verbal, will be exercised when he liaises with other services to co-ordinate care alongside the registered nurse. Demonstrating empathy is also a core skill as building trust is premised to ensuring Tyler co-operates and an open discussion is promoted.

Activity 4.4 Critical thinking (page 66)

- Patient goals

Goals enable patients, carers, and the multidisciplinary team to identify what primary concerns there are. The purpose of goal planning is to allow those involved (multidisciplinary team, patients and carers) to focus on strengths and enable the patient/client to achieve their goals in relation to health and well-being. As a nursing associate, while you will not provide a diagnosis, you will be identifying what the primary concerns are. This will then formulate the goals alongside the registered nurse. It is important to remember and refer to the *Standards of Proficiencies for Nursing Associates*, so you continually work within your parameters of practice. During the assessment, Mohammed may have identified a short-term goal for Tyler and that is to attend the GP surgery for an asthma review.

- Planning

After identifying patient goals, a care plan will be devised to instruct who will meet specific identified goals. For Tyler's care plan, while as a nursing associate you will identify primary needs, care planning will need to be discussed in conjunction with the registered nurse. Here recognition of who will be involved in meeting Tyler's needs will be discussed. Referrals to other services will be made. Each organisation will have its own specific care plan tool that will be utilised for patients. Therefore it is advisable to familiarise yourself with the care plans used in that organisation. The purpose of planning will also need to include the individual responsible, time frame and when it will be reviewed.

- Implementation

During this stage nursing associates and other key MDT/interprofessional team members will action the goals identified.

- Evaluation

After each goal has been actioned, it will be reviewed within a timely manner indicated on the care plan. There may be instances where goals may be reviewed before the given time frame indicated. This may be due to a variety of factors and directed by the patient/ client or MDT/interprofessional team member. It is important to remember goals can be added and evaluated during the patient's/client's care as at every contact patients will be assessed to add or review goals.

Further reading

NHS (2019) *NHS Long Term Plan*. Available at www.longtermplan.nhs.uk/

The plan sets out key ambitions for the NHS over ten years. Main clinical priorities include service improvement for cancer, cardiovascular disease, maternity and neonatal health, mental health, stroke, diabetes and respiratory care. All these clinical priorities have been chosen for their impact on the population's health.

NHS (2014) *Five Year Forward View*. Available at www.england.nhs.uk/wp-content/ uploads/2014/10/5yfv-web.pdf

Published in 2014 it sets out the vision for the future of the NHS. The purpose of the publication was to recognise why change was needed, what that change might look like and how services will need to achieve it.

NHS (2016) *The Five Year Forward View for Mental Health*. Available at www.england. nhs.uk/wp-content/uploads/2016/02/Mental-Health-Taskforce-FYFV-final.pdf

This plan sets out a blueprint to achieve key changes to improve mental health outcomes across the NHS. The approach identifies three key areas that need to be implemented to deliver real change.

Care Act 2014 c.23. Available at www.legislation.gov.uk/ukpga/2014/23/contents/enacted

The Act sets out duties and responsibilities for local authorities about care and support for adults who need support without delays.

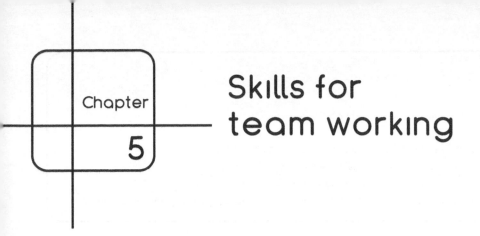

Skills for team working

NMC STANDARDS OF PROFICIENCY FOR NURSING ASSOCIATES

This chapter will address the following platforms and proficiencies:

Platform 3: Provide and monitor care

At the point of registration, the registered nursing associate will be able to:

3.7 demonstrate and apply an understanding of how and when to escalate to the appropriate professional for expert help and advice

3.4 demonstrate the knowledge, communication and relationship management skills required to provide people, families and carers with accurate information that meets their needs before, during and after a range of interventions

Platform 4: Working in teams

At the point of registration, the registered nursing associate will be able to:

4.1 demonstrate an awareness of the roles, responsibilities, and scope of practice of different members of the nursing and interdisciplinary team, and their role within it

4.2 demonstrate an ability to support and motivate other members of the care team and interact confidently with them

4.5 demonstrate an ability to prioritise and manage their own workload, and recognise where elements of care can safely be delegated to other colleagues, carers, and family members

4.6 demonstrate the ability to monitor and review the quality of care delivered, providing challenge and constructive feedback, when an aspect of care has been delegated to others

Platform 6: Contributing to integrated care

At the point of registration, the registered nursing associate will be able to:

6.1 understand the roles of the different providers of health and care. Demonstrate the ability to work collaboratively and in partnership with professionals from different agencies in interdisciplinary teams

6.6 demonstrate an understanding of their own role and contribution when involved in the care of a person who is undergoing discharge or a transition of care between professionals, settings, or services

Skills for
Chapter aims

After reading this chapter, you should be able to:

- discuss the skills required for effective prioritisation and delegation;
- effectively communicate when providing feedback, mentoring and coaching;
- understand working as a team and sharing a vision;
- understand professional roles and boundaries, lines of responsibility and reporting mechanisms.

Introduction

Healthcare professionals are required to work as a team by the nature of the role and the environment in which they work. Caring for patients in a compassionate, person-centred way is a team activity. It relies on staff who work together in any department or ward area to work effectively together. It is essential to understand the importance of teamwork and the positive impact good team working has on the quality of care experienced by patients but also the experience and motivation of staff.

A team can be made of highly skilled individuals practising within their own sphere of competence with knowledge and skills, but for patients and service users to benefit fully, there needs to be good collaboration with one another. Prioritising and delegation of tasks, effective and clear communication, and holding a shared vision with a clear understanding of everyone's roles and responsibilities is paramount for good team working. An open and honest culture that includes constructive feedback and role-modelling behaviours, the ability to question and ask for help without being concerned it portrays a lack of ability is key to reducing stress and work overload and reducing the risks of errors and harm.

Team working has been discussed at length in Chapters 3 and 4, but what skills are required for effective team working? How can we as healthcare professionals develop these skills to implement in practice?

This chapter will encourage you to consider your knowledge and skills in relation to issues of accountability in a professionally regulated role. It will encourage you to critically reflect on situations in practice and areas for improvement and the impact on patient and staff experience. You will be encouraged to consider your own practice and identify areas of improvement and your role in the development of others through providing constructive feedback and role-modelling professional behaviours.

Prioritisation, time management and delegation

Prioritising workload

When faced with what feels like a never-ending task list it is easy to choose to prioritise tasks that can be accomplished quickly and with fewest resources. This reduces the overwhelming feeling of having lots of tasks to complete. Prioritisation, however, takes into account what tasks need to be completed as a priority rather than the easiest and quickest to achieve: it can be identified what can be managed at a later date and also what tasks can be delegated.

At its core, prioritisation is based on Maslow's Hierarchy of Needs theory (1943), and healthcare professionals view activities in terms of how urgent or important they are. These decisions are based on both critical thinking and their clinical decision-making skills (Aggar et al., 2017).

Maslow's Hierarchy of Needs theory is essentially five levels to prioritise an individual's needs from highest to lowest priority. The five levels are:

1. Basic physiological need

For example, gastrointestinal needs such as foods, fluid, nutrition as well as elimination. Respiratory status and effort or cardiovascular stability or health.

2. Safety and security

For example, preventing further injury or subsequent illness.

3. Love and belonging

For example, ensuring adequate support systems are in place and maintained. This can prevent feelings of loneliness and isolation.

4. Self-esteem

For example, building a positive outlook, establishing control, and promoting a sense of worthiness.

5. Self-actualisation

For example, the full development of an individual's abilities and appreciation for life. Self-actualised people have an acceptance of who they are despite their faults and limitations.

Activity 5.1 Prioritisation

Matthew is 46 years old and had open heart surgery less than 24 hours ago.

As the nursing associate caring for Matthew, think about the order in which the following concerns/tasks should be prioritised. What is your rationale and how do they fit in the hierarchy of needs?

A. Matthew is very concerned about how his sternal incision scar will look once it is healed and is asking to talk about this and long-term options for scar management.
B. Matthew's care plan states he needs physiotherapy to commence to mobilise him – the referral needs to be made.
C. Matthew has mottled and cool upper and lower extremities. The capillary refill time is 4–5 seconds.
D. You need to complete teaching with Matthew regarding sternal precautions to prevent complications.
E. Matthew's wife has not visited since his surgery because Matthew has told her not to come as he doesn't want her to see him unwell as she will get upset.

An outline answer is provided at the end of the chapter.

Time management

Effective time management is an essential skill for all healthcare professionals. The benefits of good time management are that, essentially, we can get more done in the time we have. It can produce a higher quality of work and ensures that tasks are not missed. From an individual perspective it can also limit burn-out and improve both our professional and personal job satisfaction. But effective time management takes practice and experience. It needs to be developed. As healthcare professionals we need to find the right resources, tools and role models to help us in successful and effective time management.

Activity 5.2   Reflection

How effective are you at time management?

Take some time to reflect on your time management skills. Think about your personal life as well as your professional role.

- What strategies or tools do you use in your time management? Think about the other team members you work with.
- Can you identify a healthcare professional you work with who has good time management skills? Try to identify things they do that you think would help you in future practice.
- Think about an experience in practice when you feel you could have managed your time more effectively. What could you have done differently?

As this activity is based on your own reflection, no outline answer is provided at the end of this chapter.

A key principle of time management is planning and organisation: thinking logically about what activities need to be completed and how long realistically is needed to complete the activity or task. Breaking tasks down into smaller, more manageable tasks can help. It is important to always remember that things will not always go to plan. Unexpected situations or events can alter priorities and we need to be flexible and adaptable to meet the changing needs of our patients/clients and clinical areas. It is also important to be able to ask for help. Identifying that you have over-committed or don't have the capacity to safely undertake a task at that time and asking for support from more experienced healthcare professionals is vital. It should not be viewed as a weakness. Multitasking can lead to increased stress and increases the chances that errors may be made, or things missed.

Appropriate delegation of tasks is a key component in time management and an integral part of team working.

Delegation

Delegation within nursing can be described as a *dynamic process that involves responsibility, accountability and authority* (Sullivan and Decker, 2005, page 144). The art of delegation is an essential skill for any registered professional.

A task may be delegated from:

- one registered professional to another;
- a registered professional to an unregulated member of staff;
- a registered or unregistered person to a carer or family member.

Delegating a task to an unregistered healthcare professional such as a healthcare assistant, clinical support worker, nursery nurse, etc., involves you remaining accountable for the task, and the individual you delegate to assumes responsibility.

The responsibilities of nursing associates where delegation is concerned don't change in circumstances if the person delegating and the person accepting a delegated task are both registered professionals. As a registered professional, whether you are someone delegating a task, or receiving a delegated task, you are accountable for your conduct and practice.

For someone to be accountable they must:

- have the ability (knowledge and skills) to perform the activity or intervention;
- accept the responsibility for doing the activity;
- have the authority to perform the activity within their role, through delegation and the policies and protocols of the organisation.

The NMC *Code* sets out expectations of people on the register when they delegate to others. These requirements apply, regardless of who the activity is being delegated to. This may be another registered professional, a non-registered colleague, or a patient or carer. The Nursing and Midwifery Council (NMC) *Code* (2018b) states in the section entitled 'Practise effectively' that registrants must:

- only delegate tasks and duties that are within the other person's scope of competence, making sure that they fully understand the instructions;
- make sure that everyone they delegate tasks to are adequately supervised and supported so they can provide safe and compassionate care;
- confirm that the outcome of any task delegated to someone else meets the required standard.

Understanding who you are accountable to is key when delegating. As healthcare professionals we are accountable to ourselves, our peers, patients, colleagues, and our employers as well as professional bodies.

Read the case study below and consider the different levels of accountability for the individuals involved.

Case study: Suzanna

Suzanna is a nursing associate working on a busy paediatric surgical unit. She has four patients she is caring for in a bay. It is approaching ward round and Suzanna is prioritising the tasks she needs to complete.

Patient A has a post-operative surgical wound that the doctors have requested to review on ward round. Analgesia has been given in preparation for the dressing change, so she needs to undertake that task in a timely manner.

(Continued)

(Continued)

Patient B required hourly blood glucose levels monitoring. Mum is very anxious that these are undertaken on time and is asking when Suzanna intends on completing the task.

Patient C requires vital signs recorded and has been having pyrexias that may require further investigation. The last temperature was recorded as 38.2 but it was too early to give antipyretics. The temperature needs to be checked and if necessary, medication administered and appropriate escalation.

Patient D is due a routine set of observations.

Karl is the healthcare assistant on the ward. He offers to help. Karl usually works on an adult outpatients' unit but has been on the ward a number of times before. Suzanna assesses the situation and the tasks that she needs to complete. She asks Karl what experience he has and what tasks he is comfortable and competent to undertake. He explains that he has undertaken vital signs on children numerous times and has had teaching from the trust specific to paediatrics. He has seen blood glucose monitoring being undertaken and has done the procedure himself before under supervision. This was in an adult area and the equipment appears different, but he is happy to do this. He doesn't have much experience in wound care but feels he can take the dressing down for review.

Suzanna makes the decision that her priority is to check the blood glucose level. She will undertake this as she feels Karl is not competent in the skill and familiar with the equipment, and Mum's anxiety means she may need to spend some time with the family. She checks when the analgesia was given for the dressing change on Patient A and ascertains that she has some flexibility, and requests with the nurse in charge that the patient be seen last on ward round to allow her time to undertake the dressing in preparation. Suzanna asks Karl to undertake vital signs monitoring on the remaining patients. She gives him specific instructions as to what vital signs must be undertaken and recorded, and that she needs to be made aware of any recordings outside of the normal range or changes in the patient trend. She specifically asks him to inform her of what temperature he records for Patient C as soon as he has completed and documented it.

She finishes the conversation by checking with Karl that he is clear on what she has asked him to undertake, and he knows what information she needs from him when the tasks are completed.

Suzanna records Patient B's blood glucose level and reassures Mum. She then begins to undertake the dressing change on Patient A when Karl arrives to let her know that the vital signs have all been recorded and documented: paediatric early warning score is 0 and Patient C's temperature is 36.8. He has already informed the doctors of this as they arrived to review the patient while he was undertaking the observations. Suzanna thanks him and completes the dressing removal in preparation for review.

Activity 5.3   Critical Thinking

It is important that delegation takes into account the individual context of every situation and does not just focus on the activities required. Reading the case study above, consider Suzanna's decisions and critical thinking in the choices she has made. Think about the following questions and evaluate whether Suzanna delegated and prioritised appropriately.

- Is delegation in the best interests of the patient?
- Has Suzanna considered the clinical risk involved in delegating?

- Did Karl have the capacity to take on additional work?
- Does Karl have the skills and knowledge required to undertake the activity, including communication and interpersonal skills, as well as clinical competence?

An outline answer is provided at the end of this chapter.

Communication and providing feedback

Patient safety experts agree that communication and teamwork skills are essential for providing quality healthcare. When all clinical and non-clinical staff collaborate effectively, healthcare teams can improve patient outcomes, prevent medical errors, improve efficiency and increase patient satisfaction. Good teamwork requires effective communication, leadership, situational awareness and mutual support. Providing feedback and supporting all members of the team is an integral part of developing leadership skills in the profession. There are various models of support used in the clinical setting that involve providing feedback, and communication skills are a key element of all of them. This support can come from any member of the team and developing skills to effectively offer feedback that is received and interpreted in the right way is paramount.

Used in the correct way and with intent, feedback and coaching can accelerate clinical learning. Coaching is a partnership between the coach and another individual. The coach helps the individual to achieve their personal best and to produce the results they want in their personal and professional lives. Coaching ensures the individual can give their best, learn and develop in the way they wish.

Coaching tends to involve the development of competency, and results in motivation from developing skills in a task as the product (Bach and Ellis, 2011). Mentoring is more involved in role modelling and has subtle differences such as mentoring has a greater interest in the individual's progress and personal growth rather than simply being able to undertake a required skill.

In whatever form feedback is delivered, it takes an amount of self-awareness and effective communication skills to ensure that the intent of the feedback is the same as the impact it has on the individual receiving it. Positive feedback can result in motivation, an increase in confidence and positively influence future practice. If the feedback includes areas for improvement or identification of a mistake, for example, individuals can easily feel criticised and become defensive, and this can result in conflict within teams that, if not managed appropriately, can result in a breakdown of relationships and ineffective teamwork.

The case study below demonstrates how effective communication can result in positive outcomes for those involved and providing feedback can have a positive influence on practice and individuals.

Case study: Suzanna

During the interaction with Karl earlier in the day, Suzanna has identified some areas that she feels she needs to feedback and discuss further with Karl. She has reflected on the interaction and discusses it with the nurse in charge. Suzanna is concerned that Karl

(Continued)

(Continued)

appeared to be willing to undertake blood glucose monitoring on a patient despite the fact he didn't hold a competency and was unfamiliar with the equipment. Suzanna and the nurse in charge agree this needs to be addressed with Karl and agree on additional feedback that would benefit Karl and his development. They decide that Suzanna will offer Karl the feedback with the support of the nurse in charge. Suzanna finds an appropriate time in the shift when Karl is free and asks if she and the nurse in charge can speak with him. Karl looks concerned but she offers reassurances. She starts by thanking Karl for his help. He identified she was struggling with workload and offered to help, and she appreciated that. She recalls the fact he followed her instructions, documented appropriately and brought her the information she requested in the time frame she had specified. She then asks Karl some questions.

'Do you have any thoughts about why I asked you to do the vital signs for the patients rather than the blood glucose monitoring?'

Karl replies that he assumed it was because he didn't have the right experience and competence to do this point of care test. Suzanna confirms that was the reason and goes on to explain that any skill needs to be competence assessed and he needs training on the medical devices also. Karl agrees he was aware of this, has always adhered to it and misunderstood that he thought she would supervise him. He would not undertake anything he didn't have the training to do so. She comments on the fact that Karl has been doing a lot of shifts on the ward recently and asks if it is an area of interest for him. He confirms that he enjoys working on the paediatric wards and is keen to gain more experience. The nurse in charge suggests that she would be happy to discuss supporting Karl to attend any training he may be interested in that would benefit his role and support his personal and professional development.

Karl is happy with this and thanks them both for their feedback. He enjoys working on the ward and would like to consider paediatrics in the future.

Both Suzanna and the nurse in charge are satisfied that Karl is aware of his boundaries and scope of competence. Karl feels a valued member of the team and is pleased about the potential opportunities for his development.

This was a positive experience for all those involved. Suzanna feels reassured that there is no patient safety concern, and Karl has been offered some professional development opportunities and feels he has been recognised for his contributions to the team.

Sharing a vision and lines of responsibility

Workplace objectives are specific goals that an organisation or a department sets out to achieve in a specified time frame. Put another way, objectives are statements that explain how goals will be achieved. Objectives must be measurable and quantifiable; they must also be realistic and attainable within a specific time frame.

Teamwork is about striving to accomplish a set of common goals and objectives. For teams to be effective they need to have clear, shared objectives that contribute to the effectiveness of the care provided to patients and their families. These objectives provide a framework for the team to measure progress, recognise potential risk and identify opportunities for collaborative working.

Activity 5.4   Teamwork and objectives

- Consider how the work of teams can support the achievement of workplace objectives.
- Think about your own team.
- What evidence is there that you work together to meet objectives?
- Does your organisation have a 'mission statement' about team working?

As this activity is based on your own reflection, no outline answer is provided at the end of this chapter.

Teams function most efficiently when members share a common understanding of one another's roles and responsibilities. Indeed, one of the reasons why teams fail is a lack of clarity among team members regarding their respective roles, responsibilities and the expectations they hold of one another when working together to accomplish their vision, mission, goals and objectives. When roles and responsibilities are clearly defined, team members are more productive. There is less duplication of effort, less confusion, disappointment and frustration, and greater productivity. Team members look beyond their own individual positions and learn to understand, respect and value the unique contributions of one another, and they recognise that the overall success of the team is a function of shared responsibility and ownership.

Different members of the team will have different responsibilities and will contribute different skills and knowledge within the team. The extent of the team you work within will differ depending on the organisation you work for. For example, if you work in a care home that provides personal care only, the diversity of the team you work within will not be as great as if you work within a hospital. The importance of each team member being clear about both their own role and that of every other member of the team is essential. This understanding of the role should include the purpose of the role, together with the levels of accountability, authority and responsibility associated with the role. This understanding is crucial at an individual, team and organisational level for the team to function effectively. If team members are not clear about their roles and responsibilities or do not appreciate the roles of others, this can lead to conflict, so paying attention to your role and the roles of others can go a long way in reducing the risk of conflict within the team.

Depending on where you work, you may have an organisational chart that represents the structure of the organisation in terms of rank. The chart will show the managers and sub-workers who make up the organisational team, as well as the relationship between staff in the organisation. Again, this will depend on where you work and whether there are different departments within your organisation. Understanding these lines of reporting and escalation process is vital in understanding individuals' roles and responsibilities. Complete the activity below to explore your understanding of the structure of your teams.

Activity 5.5   Reflection

Explain lines of reporting and responsibility in your team. Draw a 'family tree' which represents the organisational structure of your clinical area. Explain each role and the responsibility attached to the role.

(Continued)

(Continued)

   Think about lines of reporting – who do you report and escalate to? Who escalates and reports to you?

   As this activity is based on your own reflection, no outline answer is provided at the end of this chapter.

Chapter summary

This chapter began with looking at the key skills of prioritisation and delegation, and the communication skills involved in effective team working. The effective delivery, planning and organization of care delivered depends on a wide range of individuals such as professionals, families and patients working together with the common goal of achieving the best health outcomes. Effective team working is essential to place people at the centre of care decisions. Understanding the different characteristics of teams and the individuals within them can help nursing associates to uphold professional caring values and to work effectively.

Activities: Brief outline answers

Activity 5.1 Prioritisation (page 77)

One potential answer for order of priority is:

C. Matthew has mottled and cool upper and lower extremities. The capillary refill time is 4–5 seconds – *this involves a basic physiological need, possible complication related to the cardiovascular system.*

B. Matthew's care plan states he needs physiotherapy to commence to mobilise him – the referral needs to be made – *safety and security.*

D. You need to complete teaching with the patient regarding sternal precautions to prevent complications – *safety and security.*

E. Matthew's wife has not visited since his surgery because Matthew has told her not to come as he doesn't want her to see him unwell as she will get upset – *love and belonging.*

A. Matthew is very concerned about how his sternal incision scar will look once it is healed and is asking to talk about this and long-term options for scar management – *self-esteem.*

Activity 5.3 Critical thinking (page 80)

Suzanna considered the tasks that needed to be taken and prioritised them in order of patient need. She identified the time-sensitive nature of some of the tasks and considered this when deciding that delegation was appropriate for patient care and safety. She identified that the pain relief was required for dressing change and this needed to be considered in her decision. She also identified the anxiety of the patient's mother and that she may need some support and reassurances. Suzanna also considered who would be appropriate to give that reassurance.

She carefully considered the clinical risks associated with each patient and based her clinical decision making on this.

Karl offered to help Suzanna and she accepted as she identified she was not able to undertake all the tasks, and it was in the best interests of her patients.

Suzanna identified Karl's level of competence and delegated appropriately ensuring he had clear instruction of what she needed him to do and following up on the outcomes and appropriate escalation. She identified that although he may be experienced in his usual place of work, this is a different clinical area with potentially different equipment.

Further reading

Esterhuizen, P (2019) *Reflective Practice in Nursing.* 4th edition. London: SAGE/Learning Matters.

Reflection is an essential tool for nursing associates and all registered practitioners. Developing good reflective skills on our practice and our interactions with others will help us develop as healthcare professionals.

Grant, A and Goodman, B (2019) *Communication and Interpersonal Skills in Nursing.* 4th edition. London: SAGE.

This book discusses many different perspectives of interpersonal skills and communications techniques. This will enhance the discussions in this chapter about communication and providing and receiving feedback.

Belbin, M (2012) *Team Roles at Work.* [Online]. Taylor and Francis.

This book explores the impact of team roles from interpersonal chemistry and managing difficult relationships, to cultivating effective leaders and shaping organisations. It provides insights in to how to apply the theory of team working to everyday work situations.

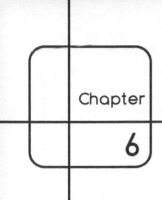

Chapter

6

How to be heard in difficult situations

NMC STANDARDS OF PROFICIENCY FOR NURSING ASSOCIATES

This chapter will address the following platforms and proficiencies:

Platform 1: Being an accountable professional

At the point of registration, the registered nursing associate will be able to:

- 1.1 understand and act in accordance with *The Code: Professional Standards of Practice and Behaviour for Nurses, Midwives and Nursing Associates* and fulfil all registration requirements
- 1.3 understand the importance of courage and transparency and apply the Duty of Candour, recognising and reporting any situations, behaviours or errors that could result in poor care outcomes
- 1.4 demonstrate an understanding of, and the ability to, challenge or report discriminatory behaviour
- 1.10 demonstrate the skills and abilities required to develop, manage and maintain appropriate relationships with people, their families, carers and colleagues

Platform 4: Working in teams

At the point of registration, the registered nursing associate will be able to:

- 4.1 demonstrate an awareness of the roles, responsibilities, and scope of practice of different members of the nursing and interdisciplinary team, and their role within it
- 4.2 demonstrate an ability to support and motivate other members of the care team and interact confidently with them
- 4.3 understand and apply the principles of human factors and environmental factors when working in teams
- 4.6 demonstrate the ability to monitor and review the quality of care delivered, providing challenge and constructive feedback, when an aspect of care has been delegated to others

Introduction

The Nursing and Midwifery Council (NMC) aspires to ensure that every registrant has the confidence to speak up and raise any matter or concern that they consider could impact on providing safe, kind and effective care. This might include witnessing or suspecting poor practice or a risk to patient safety. It is important to remember that speaking out is part of the day-to-day professional practice expected of everyone on the NMC register. But it is also important to ensure nursing and midwifery professionals feel supported if you do raise a concern.

The importance of raising concerns, and the rights of professionals to do so, is enshrined in the NMC *Code* (2018b). There are three important elements to bear in mind:

- You should act without delay if there are risks to patient safety or public protection, remembering that this may be in any setting: clinical practice, research, education, policy or management.
- You shouldn't hinder anyone else from raising a concern if they wish to do so.
- You should protect anyone for whom you have management responsibility from any unwarranted treatment if they raise a concern.

The requirements around speaking up therefore have implications for all of us, in terms of our professional duty as practising registrants, colleagues, managers or leaders.

We also know there are times when things have gone wrong, sometimes over a long period of time, where nursing and midwifery professionals have not felt able to speak up because other colleagues do not seem concerned. There are lots of possible explanations for this, such as a lack of confidence or thinking that more senior staff or other professionals know best. We know people may even fear they will be treated differently if they speak up or risk being branded a 'troublemaker'.

We have seen from past reviews and inquiries that people stop speaking up when they are not listened to, or if nothing changes in response to concerns raised. In those instances, solutions cannot be found, and risks can be left unmanaged. Staff may 'give up' or move on to new roles in an organisation where they believe there is a better safety culture in which staff will be listened to, and where learning and improvement are more valued.

So, deciding whether something really poses a risk or not, and then deciding if, when and how to speak up, is not easy and it can be stressful. However, it matters that professionals do speak out and do so in a timely way. The challenge comes for all healthcare professionals in how they can do this professionally and effectively. Developing interpersonal skills and the ability to report errors and poor practice is a key part of this, as well as understanding the environmental and human factors that influence practice and team working experiences.

This chapter will explore the environmental and human factors that influence team working and support the development of key skills to manage difficult situations and working with others.

Challenging and reporting errors: near misses and poor practice

Reporting errors and near misses

It is never easy to raise a concern or report a colleague but if you witness activity or care that poses a risk to patients you have a duty to report it. This includes not only actual errors but near misses.

There are lots of reasons why we are reluctant to report errors and near misses. We are worried about being blamed or seen as incompetent but also have concerns about being seen as a troublemaker if we report colleagues or other staff members. Working in healthcare is a safety critical activity. There are lots of opportunities when things can go wrong. People get distracted, forget to document things and adverse incidents happen. To keep our patients safe, we need to maintain a constant vigilance on how we work and the ways we work together, not be afraid to admit when we make mistakes and having honest conversations with one another.

What is meant by a near miss?

WHO defines a near miss as *an error that has the potential to cause an adverse event (patient harm) but fails to do so because of chance or because it is intercepted.* Near misses and no-harm incidents can provide valuable information, much of which cannot be captured by adverse event-reporting systems, therefore, reporting such incidents should be encouraged.

We will now explore how this might play out in practice with the following activity and the case study of Stephen.

Case study: Stephen

Stephen is working on a paediatric ward and caring for nine-year-old Holly who has been admitted with a severe throat infection and commenced on oral antibiotics. Stephen is checking the medication with his senior band 6 registered nurse on the ward.

During the checking procedure Stephen discovers that the incorrect dose has been prescribed. He identifies that this is the first dose to be given so no harm has come to Holly, but had this been given she would have received a larger dose than recommended.

Stephen contacts the prescriber and asks for the dose to be reviewed. The doctor who prescribed the medication agrees the dose prescribed was more than the recommended dose and re-prescribes the correct dose. He explained he has not worked in paediatrics very much and when prescribing for adults he is used to standard dosages.

Stephen administers the medication to Holly and documents in her medical notes that the incorrect dose was initially prescribed. He also completed an incident reporting form. He informs the doctor who prescribed the antibiotic in a professional and polite manner that he has reported the incident.

Activity 6.1   Reflection

Think about your own reporting systems in your trust or place of work. Do you know the process of escalation when a near miss has been identified?

Would have you done anything differently to Stephen in this situation?

An outline answer is provided at the end of the chapter.

Communication skills

Developing enhanced verbal communication skills is paramount to developing leadership skills and the ability to professionally escalate concerns and challenge poor behaviours and practice. Communicating accurately with an awareness of pitch, tone and volume are key in verbal communication. Developing questioning skills and the ability to present information accurately to others is also an important element.

Speaking up, or assertiveness, is a vital social skill in professional contexts and in everyday interactions, but not everyone can master this skill. It is human nature to worry about how others perceive us and our actions. Being assertive can often be viewed as being bossy or telling others what to do.

Communication is seen as a basic tool, but the quality of the communication has a strong relationship to its effectiveness. One theoretical model that helps us understand how communication takes place is the linear framework of communication (Bach and Grant, 2015).

Active listening requires full concentration on what is being said by others, without letting themselves be distracted. It serves the purpose of earning the trust of others, helping them understand the situation (Cuncic, 2019). Individuals can listen to others, however, most of the time they do not hear what is actually being said. This can be caused by thoughts that occupy our minds which distract us from listening. It's common for listeners to be tempted to want to fill a silence by asking questions right away, giving their own opinion or sharing a similar experience (Mulder, 2018). Many people also have the tendency to give advice before letting the other person finish. In addition to these listening barriers, distraction is the biggest culprit that makes it hard to listen actively sometimes. Think of thoughts that keep popping up in your head, the tendency to check our smartphones, trying to overhear other people's conversations and looking at our surroundings.

Active listening means that the speaker gets enough time and space to vent his thoughts, feelings and opinions and express himself well. When you practise active listening, you make the other person feel heard and valued. In this way, active listening is the foundation for any successful conversation.

The linear model is the simplest form of communication and involves messages being sent and received by two or more people. While this model demonstrates how communication occurs in its simplest form, it fails to consider other factors impacting on the process. Communication in nursing practice can be complicated, involving the conveyance of large amounts of information, for example, when providing patients with information relating to their care and treatment or when offering health promotion advice.

In contrast, the circular transactional model is a two-way approach, acknowledging other factors which influence communication such as feedback and validation. Successful communication is focused, purposeful and identifies the following skills: person-centred context, goal, mediating process, response, feedback and perception. It also considers other aspects of the individual and the influence these may have on their approach to the process of communication.

For communication to be effective it is important for the nursing associate to recognise key components, and intrinsic and extrinsic factors, which may affect the process. They must consider factors such as past personal experiences, personal perceptions, timing and the setting in which communication occurs. Physical, physiological, psychological and semantic noise may also influence the message, resulting in misinterpretation.

When communicating face to face, a lot of information is transmitted through non-verbal means. This makes things like telephone calls and e-mails very challenging. Communication can be even more complex when attempting to communicate across different professions, specialities or hierarchical barriers. As we don't always use the same language, have the same level of expertise or knowledge, or even have a good understanding of the other individual's role.

Poor communication is one of the leading causes of adverse incident or errors. A variety of tools to aid communication, like SBAR (Situation Background Assessment Recommendation) can be used. Find out what your organisation uses and practise its use when communicating.

Inadequate verbal and written communication is recognised as being the most common root cause of serious errors and incidents. There are some fundamental barriers to communication. These include hierarchy, gender, ethnic background and differences in communication styles between disciplines and individuals. Communication is more effective in teams where there are standard communication structures in place. This is where the use of SBAR can add real value.

SBAR takes the ambiguity out of important communications. It prevents the use of assumptions, vagueness or reticence that sometimes occur – particularly when staff are uncomfortable about making a recommendation due to inexperience or their position in the hierarchy.

It can help to prevent breakdowns in verbal and written communication by creating a shared mental model around all patient handovers and situations requiring escalation, or critical exchange of information.

Using the SBAR tool (Figure 6.1) is an effective way of levelling the traditional hierarchy between doctors and other care givers by building a common language for communicating critical events and reducing communication barriers between different healthcare professionals. It is easy to remember and encourages staff to think and prepare before communicating. This can make handovers quicker yet more effective, thereby releasing more time for clinical care.

SITUATION	My name is …
	I am a Nursing Associate on Ward … looking after "patient x"
	I am calling because …
	Example issues –
	• Change in vital signs
	• Increase in Early Warning Score
	• Increased pain
	• Parental concern (if child)

(Continued)

Figure 6.1 (Continued)

BACKGROUND	The patient was admitted on ... date with a history of ...
	Brief information regarding –
	• Investigation / procedures
	• Usual condition
	• Last set of vital signs
ASSESSMENT	I think the problem may be ...
	I have already done –
	• Administered analgesia
	• Administered oxygen
	OR
	I am concerned and the patient is deteriorating
RECOMMENDATION	The patient needs to be reviewed within ... minutes.
	What would you advise while I await your review?

Figure 6.1 The SBAR Tool (Adapted from *British Journal of Nursing* 2020, Using the SBAR handover tool)

Activity 6.2 Reflection

Think about your communication strengths and weaknesses.

Have you been in the situation where the message you intended to convey has been misinterpreted?

How did you manage the situation?

As this activity is based on your own reflection, no outline answer is given at the end of this chapter.

Challenging poor practice

As registrants on the NMC register we all have a responsibility to challenge and report poor practice. It is never easy to raise concerns about a colleague, but if you witness care or actions that pose a risk to patients, you have a duty to tackle this head on.

Being non-judgemental when you suspect poor practice is hard, as your intuition and senses have already been alerted to what you perceive as an uncomfortable situation. However, it's important that you test out what you suspect and therefore you need to put your worries to one side initially and attempt to carry out a non-judgemental observation. This means looking or listening again with a mind that is completely open. In some situations, you might wish to do this over a period of time as it can help you understand more clearly what's going on (Brewin, 2012).

Sometimes when we encounter something at work that isn't right it's possible to point out the mistake there and then in a way that isn't confrontational. We call this challenging in the moment. For most people who have been thoughtless but not intentionally negligent, this type of interaction should be enough to get them to realise the inappropriateness of their action and change their behaviour.

Consider how this might play out in the following scenario.

Case study: Mrs Lees

Two of your colleagues are helping some residents with their lunch. They are sat at the table with three residents but are discussing their evening out together and not interacting appropriately with the residents. You notice that one of the residents, Mrs Lees, is trying to reach her water but can't. The two staff members seem unaware and engrossed in their conversation.

You decide to address this with your colleagues directly by politely letting them know that Mrs Lees would like a drink, and asking if they can help her reach for the water: 'Hi Sarah, I think Mrs Lees would like a drink. She's trying to reach her water, can you help her? Why don't you talk about your night out on your coffee break? I am sure Mrs Lee would much rather hear about Mrs Cain's visit from her daughter. She brought her some lovely flowers'.

Addressing this at the time and in a non-threatening way should be enough to change their actions.

Sometimes challenging in the moment just doesn't work. You may have tried it, but the poor practice continues. Or it could be that the situation you've encountered is just too serious to deal with in this way. If this is the case, you need to go to your manager and bring the poor practice to their attention. We will now explore how this might work in practice through the case study of Shumira, and the following activity.

Case study: Shumira

Shumira is a nursing associate who works on a trauma and orthopaedic ward. She has worked on the ward for around six months and feels part of the team. She has built good working relationships with the staff.

Amanda is a senior health care assistant who has worked on the ward for ten years or more. She is well respected and popular with the team, and is seen as hardworking and a team player.

Amanda asks Shumira to help her get Mr Lawson out of bed. Shumira is happy to help and follows Amanda to the room. Shumira recalls from handover that Mr Lawson's risk assessment details that a hoist should be used for transfer, so she tells Amanda she is going to get the equipment. Amanda tells her that the hoist is out of service, so she plans to get Mr Lawson out of bed without it.

Shumira is uncomfortable with this and clearly tells Amanda that it is unsafe to do the transfer without the correct equipment and she is not happy to help her. She checks that Mr Lawson is comfortable and tells Amanda she is going to try to find a hoist from somewhere else or speak to the physio for further guidance. When she returns to the room Mr Lawson is sat in his chair.

She finds Amanda who tells her rather rudely that she got one of the other healthcare assistants to help her as Shumira couldn't be bothered. She doesn't appear to understand what Shimura's issue is – she has done it this way before and no one else seems to mind. Shumira wants to avoid an argument with Amanda who is clearly annoyed. She simply tells Amanda that she is concerned that the handling technique of Mr Lawson was poor practice and that she is concerned that harm could have come to Mr Lawson, but also Amanda and her colleague due to poor handling techniques not in line with the risk assessment.

Shumira escalates the incident verbally to her senior nurse in charge. The nurse in charge agrees with Shumira's assessment of the situation and Shumira is asked to complete the trust incident reporting documentation. She does this and documents in the medical notes after asking for Mr Lawson to be reviewed by the team. She also informs the physio and asks for another risk assessment to be completed.

Activity 6.3   Reflection

Review the case study above and reflect on the following questions:

- How has Shumira demonstrated good communication?
- Shumira has demonstrated courage in this situation. Identify some aspects of this that may have caused you difficulty in acting how Shumira did
- How did Shumira show competence in this situation?
- How did Shumira show commitment in this scenario?
- What could have been Shumira's next steps if the nurse in charge did not share her concerns about the incident?

An outline answer is provided at the end of this chapter.

What Shumira did in this situation showed courage. It is not always easy to challenge or speak up in situations like this.

Factors that influence ability to speak up

Sometimes you might find it easier to speak up than at other times, and there are a variety of factors which influence the ability to speak to do this. These are both individual and situational.

Individual

- *Confidence in personal knowledge* – The more staff trust their judgement the more likely they are to report poor care
- *Personal control* – Perceptions of autonomy at work can improve the likelihood of speaking up
- *Communication skills* – The ability and confidence to speak assertively and critically is important for speaking up and can be learnt
- *Severity of (perceived) risk* – The higher the perception of the potential harm to patients the greater the likelihood of reporting
- *Nature of the concerns* – Some studies suggest that health professionals are more likely to speak up about traditional threats to patient safety (e.g. staffing and equipment shortages or organisational disruption) than about a colleague's unprofessional behaviour or substandard performance
- *Perceptions of effectiveness of speaking up* – When health professionals believe their concerns will be acted on they are more likely to report

Situational factors

- *National context* – Government policy, media coverage, the action of interest groups, ethical codes and guidelines promoted by professional bodies, and the care standards expected by national regulators all affect willingness to speak up and how people respond

- *Reliance on colleagues for educational or professional advancement* – This can be a powerful inhibitor of speaking up
- *Managerial cultures and competencies* – Confidence that an organisation will respond affects decisions about speaking up

Team working and managing difficult situations

Professor Michael West's research on team-based working in healthcare suggests that care outcomes, innovation and staff retention can all be enhanced, and staff sickness, absence, stress and injury reduced, by making sure the following three features are present in your teams:

1.   A small number of meaningful objectives

A set of compelling objectives that your team members share responsibility – and accountability – for achieving, helps to create a sense of shared purpose, trust and collective achievement.

2.   Clear roles and responsibilities among team members

Team members need to be clear about what activities need to be undertaken and who is responsible for completing them, so that nothing slips through the gaps. This is especially important when teams are forming, but roles and responsibilities may shift as your team matures and you get to know one another's strengths. These roles and responsibilities should be revisited regularly to ensure that expectations about how things would work are indeed how they are working.

3.   Reflect on how the team is working together

All teams benefit from taking time out to reflect on how they are working together and how they might improve. You might want to do this in the form of team time-outs, away days or regular huddles, covering both technical aspects of work, and how people are feeling. This time will be wasted, however, if people don't feel able to contribute freely, regardless of their role or position in the management hierarchy. So it's important to think about how you will create a safe environment for your colleagues to speak up.

Activity 6.4   Reflection

- Can you think of a situation when team working wasn't very effective?
- How was it handled?
- On reflection what could have been done differently?
- Have you learnt anything from this situation?

Consider things such as:

- Was there a power gradient in this situation?
- Was it resolved to everyone's satisfaction?
- What was the impact of the conflict on the team members?

As this activity is based on your own personal experience, no outline answer is provided at the end of this chapter.

Hierarchy

Within any team there needs to be a power gradient and hierarchy. The leader is at the top as the person co-ordinating, directing and making decisions. However, this should not be absolute. If this gradient is too steep, then the leader's decisions become unquestionable, and followers simply blindly follow instructions. This is unsafe as everyone has the potential to make a mistake. Safe practice is achieved when everyone feels they can raise concerns and are able to question instructions. It is important for those in a position of hierarchy to invite people's thoughts and concerns, especially around patient safety issues. It is also important for everyone to learn how to raise concerns and challenge hierarchy appropriately.

One method that can be used to raise concerns appropriately is PACE (Probe, Alert, Challenge, Emergency). This method can be used to escalate until a satisfactory response is reached.

Probe: This can be used when someone notices something they think could be a problem. It is often verbalised as a question. 'I think you need to know what is happening here'

Alert: The statement is more direct and strengthened. A course of action can be suggested. 'I think something bad might happen'

Challenge: Urgent attention required. 'I know something bad will happen if we don't do something'

Emergency: A critical event is about to happen. 'I will not let this happen'

(Adapted from ALSG, 2016)

Emotional intelligence and team working

In 1995, Daniel Goleman published his book, *Emotional Intelligence*. Researchers who study high-performing teams were especially interested in the value of emotional intelligence. Interpersonal skills involve activities associated with the emotions of other people.

Conflict resolution in teams often requires a significant amount of emotional intelligence, especially in high-pressure or deadline roles. With each member often working to feed work back into other members of the team, even simple conflicts can create bottlenecks and stop work. Emotional intelligence greatly benefits communication skills, giving employees better tools to discuss problems empathically, to consider the other person's side, and to vent frustrations and concerns before they become major problems.

Teams should be able to work together as a cohesive whole, meaning that they should know what each is capable of in terms of time, emotional and physical energy, and quality output. Building team trust is one key factor here.

While good emotional intelligence is often about how you interact with others, it's also about how you understand yourself. Individuals who are aware of their own emotions, problems and reactions are much more likely to regulate emotions, take breaks to manage stress and react empathically when someone in their team is venting or stressed.

Emotional intelligence means recognising the efforts and input of others, which often requires action. Emotionally intelligent teams work to recognise one another's accomplishments, give credit, and are therefore often more motivated with a better sense of purpose.

Good emotional intelligence gives teams the foundation to work together productively by creating a shared sense of empathy, ensuring that team members understand one another and their problems. It allows the team to prioritise communication and collaboration.

Chapter summary

This chapter has built on some of the discussions in previous chapters around team working and communication skills. We have discussed some of the interpersonal skills required to challenge and report errors, near misses, serious incidents and poor practice, and identified some of the factors that can influence our abilities to do this.

Understanding the environmental and human factors that influence team working is an essential part of developing the required assertiveness skills needed to manage working with others and difficult situations.

Activities: Brief outline answers

Activity 6.1 Reflection (page 90)

Stephen has followed his trust policy on reporting of near misses. His reasoning for reporting the incident was not to attribute blame or get anyone into trouble – he identified there may be an educational need and this needs to be highlighted to prevent any future or actual harm.

He was polite and professional.

Activity 6.3 Reflection (page 94)

- How has Shumira demonstrated good communication?

Shumira prevented getting into a situation of conflict with Amanda, stating only the facts but in a respectful and calm way.
She documented all actions and concerns appropriately.
Escalated in a professional manner.
Included MDT members in information sharing e.g. physio.

- Shumira has demonstrated courage in this situation. Identify some aspects of this that may have caused you difficulty in acting how Shumira did.

Amanda is a popular team member who has worked on the ward for a long time. It is understandable that someone may be reluctant to challenge someone like this. Not being on the ward long herself, it takes confidence in your own knowledge to act in this way.

Amanda stated that she has done the transfer this way before and no one else minds – this could cause doubt that Shumira is correct in her objections. If no one else minds, then maybe I have got this wrong?

- How did Shumira show competence in this situation?

Shumira was aware of the risk assessment, where she could find it and the correct process to follow.

- How did Shumira show commitment in this scenario?

Shumira did not ignore what she had been made aware of – she followed through in a difficult situation, following process and her duty of care.

- What could have been Shumira's next steps if the nurse in charge did not share her concerns about the incident?

Do you know your escalation process in your trust/clinical ward area?
    Shumira could have escalated to the ward manger or senior nurse if needed. Patient safety nurse?

Further reading

Blom, L et al. (2015) The SBAR model for communication between health care professionals: a clinical intervention pilot study. *International Journal of Caring Sciences*, 8(3): 530.

The aim of this study is to evaluate hospital-based healthcare professionals' experiences from using the Situation, Background, Assessment and Recommendation (SBAR) communication model.

Bylund, C and Brown, R (2010) Theoretical models of communication skills training, in *Handbook of Communication in Oncology and Palliative Care*. Oxford: Oxford University Press.

This text provides a more in-depth look at communication models and the implementation in practice.

Nemeth, CP (2008) The context for improving healthcare team communication, in *Improving Healthcare Team Communication*. 1st edition. Routledge. pages 1–7.

This chapter uses the aviation model as a basis for reviewing healthcare communication and associated risks.

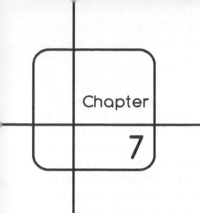

Chapter

7

Maintaining your sense of identity and resilience as a nursing associate

Chapter aims

After reading this chapter, you should be able to:

* explore the importance of self-care and seeking support in healthcare;
* explain some of the benefits of using self-care strategies when working in clinical practice;
* understand the concept of emotional intelligence and the impact of this when working with patients and team;
* identify how 'burnout' can impact on emotional and physical well-being;
* identify your resilience strategy.

Introduction

Working within healthcare means that you will encounter multiple stressors, daily practical dilemmas alongside the ever-changing emotional demands as part of your role. The recent COVID-19 pandemic has further challenged our mental health and well-being like never before. The changes that have occurred has meant a big shift in the way we work and how we approach the demands of our job. This chapter will allow you to navigate through and provide you with an understanding of why self-care is important. This will be undertaken by delving into concepts such as resilience, emotional intelligence and the impact of these in response to daily stressors as part of your role. As healthcare workers, your focus is centred around meeting the physical, social and emotional needs of the patients and families that you provide care for. This means, at times giving care under extremely emotionally intense conditions and in complex environments. The COVID-19 pandemic has been an example of how as healthcare workers there has been a need to deliver care and meet organisational targets under pressure in a continual changing healthcare landscape. This brings its own challenges as the role of the healthcare worker is associated with compassion in healthcare, but what impact does this have on healthcare workers caring for themselves in a role that is both physically and emotionally demanding? Can applying the concept of self-care reduce levels of stress, burnout, and attrition from the profession? The following chapter will allow you to explore how resilience can be maintained without losing the identity of your profession as providers of high-quality safe and compassionate care.

In 2021 the NHS employed 1.3 million people in England and there were 1.65 million jobs in adult social care which accounted for 8.6 per cent of the working age population (NHS Digital 2022). With such a percentage accounting for the NHS workforce, the health and well-being of society is dependent upon the commitment of our healthcare workforce. This has been more prevalent during the pandemic whereby healthcare workers have gone above and beyond through goodwill to provide quality of care to patients. As a nursing associate you have a professional duty as *The Code* (NMC, 2018b) states *you must maintain the level of health you need to carry out your professional role*. This means having the ability to recognise and implement strategies to maintain your mental health, to cope with stress, and acknowledge how your own feelings and emotions guide your thinking and actions.

What is stress?

Stress is a term that is used often within healthcare to describe feelings of being overwhelmed with workload (demands of the job) with diminishing resources available (to undertake the job). While stress is common within modern work organisations, nursing, which is the largest healthcare profession, has been universally described as a stressful career choice. The impact of stress on healthcare workers is well documented in literature, however, there are many factors that directly influence how an individual will react to work-related stress. As a nursing associate, you and a colleague may be providing care to a patient under the same intense conditions and under considerable pressure, but how you respond to the patient and the direct impact on you may differ. For the following activity you are required to identify and consider the factors involved in workplace stress; this will include factors such as job and individual characteristics that directly impact on how an individual responds to stress. The *Nursing Job Stress Model* conceptualised by Zeller and Levin (2013) has been adapted below to guide you in completing the activity.

Activity 7.1   Reflection

Critically think about the individual and workplace factors involved which have a psychological and physical health impact on an individual during stress.

Use the adapted guide below to complete the activity. I have added some factors in the boxes below to help.

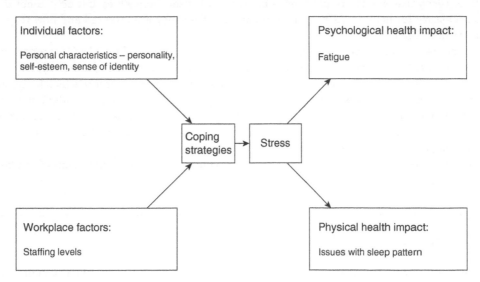

An outline answer has been provided at the end of the chapter.

The above activity would have allowed you to start thinking about the effects of stress on an individual's physical and mental health. While completing the activity you may have been able to identify with some of the factors which you may have experienced yourself. Later in the chapter you will have the opportunity to explore coping responses to workplace situations by exploring the concept of resilience.

Workplace stress can cause:

- inability to focus;
- inability to think clearly;
- inattentiveness can lead to medication and other errors;
- injury such as needle stick injuries;
- direct impact on patient care and outcomes– poor quality of care, poor patient safety, patient negative experience (dissatisfaction);
- organisation impact– worker stress will mean increased absenteeism, staff turnover, decreased productivity.

Workplace stress can also lead to burnout and compassion fatigue. Self-compassion in nursing has been described as *being receptive to one's feelings that cause suffering and hardship, approaching one's feelings with concern and warmth* (Senyuva et al., 2013). Working within the health profession we are taught to put our patients first, a notion instilled through education and training. While this is a fundamental aspect of our roles, should this be at a detriment to oneself? In everyday practice, regardless of the field of nursing you practise within as a nursing associate, you will witness situations that at times may be traumatic, ethically challenging and distressing. During these times, patients and families you care for will take priority and your feelings of being overwhelmed and exhaustion will not be an area of focus. Why do you think, as a nursing associate, this may not be an area of focus? In nursing education, we are taught skills to recognise when patients need support to look after themselves, but do you not think it is necessary for healthcare workers to recognise when they are stressed and how they can support themselves?

The concept compassion fatigue has been described because of prolonged and intense contact with patients suffering, where providing compassionate care is exceeded by the individual's ability to prioritise the self. This is usually evident in highly stressed environments in which individuals work. Prevention of compassion fatigue can be achieved through many ways including increasing compassion for self, through setting professional boundaries, self-care and self-awareness. But how easy is it to implement these prevention strategies to avoid compassion fatigue? Barriers to self-compassion can be related to internal and external factors.

Read the case study below and reflect on what you think is preventing Hanna from being compassionate to herself during times of stress.

Case study: Hanna

Hanna has been working on the dementia unit for 18 months since she qualified as a nursing associate. Prior to this she had been employed as a healthcare assistant for two years on the same ward. She had a lifelong ambition of caring for the elderly which was influenced by her grandmother who she cared for when she was receiving treatment for cancer. She was her sole carer and looked after her until she passed away three years ago. Hanna has always been an enthusiastic individual, willing to extend her shifts at work when the unit is short staffed. Since Hanna qualified, she has witnessed the hospital undergoing many changes, one being a closure of some units due to staff shortages. This was a temporary measure until staff shortages were resolved; however, this has been ongoing for the last 12 months. Hanna has been told by her manager that her current increased patient allocation will be reviewed, and support will be put in place. Hanna has been struggling with patient care as she is not being able to spend time with her patients as she would like. This frustration is impacting on her anxiety. She gets overwhelmed with her elderly dementia patients asking her to sit and spend time with them but is unable to. She recalls memories of her grandmother and the reasons why she chose healthcare as a profession. Hanna is tired all the time and is spending most of her free time sleeping which has impacted on her relationships with others. She is unable to focus on work but carries on because everyone on the unit is experiencing the same as her.

While reading this case study you may have considered some of the following internal and external barriers that Hanna is experiencing, which is preventing her from being compassionate to herself.

Internal barriers

Professional identity

In nursing, professional identity is related to how you perceive yourself and in relationship with others. This is influenced by the norms and values of the discipline and will result in how you think, act and feel. If we look at this in relation to self-compassion and your profession as a nursing associate, *The Code* (2018b) states you must uphold the standards and values set out in *The Code*; this includes treating people with compassion and responding compassionately to their needs. *The Code* (2018b) also states *You must maintain the level of health you need to carry out your professional role*. You may wonder why these two specific standards have been mentioned side by side. You will agree that to care for others compassionately you must care for yourself. However, this is not always easy when the professional identity of a healthcare worker is *hardwired to be caregivers*. Andrews et al. (2020) explore the concept of *hardwired to be caregivers* and argue nursing identity and sense of self are intertwined. The ability for one to accept caring for themselves wholly depended on how nursing identity is perceived. One of the barriers that prevents individuals from giving permission to look after their self-care is dependent on the lack of nursing education around this subject and workplace cultures that do not prioritise self-care and being compassionate to the self.

Character

Hanna is young, early in her career and relates her passion of wanting to care for others stemming from her personal experiences. The mental and physical exhaustion she is experiencing is being overlooked by her due to her relationship with others on the unit and accepting unreasonable demands because of this. Often when individuals are caught in situations where the emotional impact is high, it can be difficult to do anything else but to plough on and reach the end. This can create a negative cycle where exhaustion, frustration and anxiety make it difficult to think about a situation and how to manage the demands of the workload.

External barriers

Environment /culture

Cultures within organisations impact on how staff respond to and react to stressful working situations. In the case study, Hanna has expressed her concerns about her workload to her manager but it does not seem there has been an outcome to the concerns raised. A report by the Kings Fund (2021) explored the necessity of compassionate leadership to enable nurturing cultures within healthcare, a culture where staff are encouraged to speak up when they see things going wrong. While NHS organisations have a formal structure to raise concerns through Freedom to Speak Up Guardians, there is no equivalent for adult social care. Are you aware of Freedom to Speak Up Guardians in your area of practice? Compassionate leadership in the report is described as *leaders listening with fascination to those they lead, arriving at shared (rather than imposed) understanding of the challenges they face*. The ability to employ empathetic listening to staff concerns and valuing their views can only help and support staff that need 'permission' to acknowledge their own self-care needs.

Organisational demands

Constant changes within the NHS and organisations you work within can leave a de-stabilising effect on staff. An example of this can be restructuring of a service: during these times, staff self-care may not be a priority as the impacts of service re-structuring will take priority. One of the biggest barriers that adds to this are operational targets that come at the expense of quality of care, staff and patient experience.

Working conditions across all settings – in primary, secondary, mental health, community and social care – need to ensure support is embedded from an organisational level to combat the ever-increasing exodus of staff leaving healthcare. This means that organisations need to embed changes to the workplace that impact on health and well-being rather than tackling the issues when they become a problem. To understand this better, the report *The Courage of Compassion* (The Kings Fund 2021) sets out the ABC framework for staff to help them better understand what core needs they need to recognise to minimise workplace stress they encounter. It is important to remember this approach requires a level of self-awareness. While the framework explores core needs of the nurse and midwife, this is adaptable to nursing associates who have a key role in the healthcare team.

A – Autonomy

This looks at staff having control over their work life and to be able to act consistently with their values.

While the framework suggests key areas that need to satisfy autonomy as a core need such as influencing decision making in how care is delivered and sustaining just and fair psychological cultures, the key area that is of particular interest is staff autonomy over working schedules and conditions. Ask yourself as a nursing associate if you were involved in shared decision making about working conditions such as staff rest opportunities during work, flexibility in work schedules. Will this have a direct impact on your ability to cope?

B – Belonging

This looks at the concept of being 'connected' to and cared for by colleagues. Do you feel valued, respected and supported?

The core work needs that belonging explores are that of team working, culture and leadership. Ask yourself is team well-being an important feature of your team? Does the shared objective of team well-being feature as a core need in your workplace environment? Shared objectives within a team are usually reinforced by compassionate leadership. Therefore, does the leadership structure in your organisation nurture cultures and encourage compassionate leadership whereby staff support is a priority?

C – Contribution

This looks at areas of practice where you experience how your contribution can deliver valued outcomes. This can be influenced by a variety of factors that are essential to feel effective at work. Does management provide the opportunity for personal reflection, mentorship, and supervision so you are able to thrive at work. Do you have the opportunity to undertake development that continues personal and professional growth?

The above three core needs are the starting point for organisations to consider which contribute to staff well-being. Embedding these components within the culture of the organisation will play a key role for staff to thrive at work.

Impacts of stress – burnout

Concept of burnout

Exhaustion is an experience healthcare practitioners can often feel at the end of a shift and if it continues over time, we can shut down our awareness of what we feel, running on empty. You may find when working with others you are able to pick up on others' feelings and want to help by unconsciously taking on their energies. This makes us prone to 'burnout' if we don't learn to clear our energy field. Burnout is a term that as a healthcare practitioner you may or may not have experienced. It is difficult for everyone to be around someone who is in a burnout state, as the person seems to have lost the ability to care and connect with self and therefore others.

Burnout

The term burnout was introduced by Freudenberger in 1974 when he observed a loss of motivation and reduced commitment among volunteers at a mental health clinic (Dal'Ora et al., 2020). This concept was then further developed by Maslach in 1981 who created a scale, the Maslach Burnout Inventory (MBI), which internationally is the most widely used instrument to measure burnout. Burnout is identified as a *state of fatigue or frustration that resulted from professional relationships that failed to produce the expected results* (Freudenberger, 1974). Since this definition there have been evolving definitions of the concept which have further gone to focus on the diminished sense of personal accomplishment amongst professionals who work with other people in challenging situations. Burnout is likely to have a direct impact on quality of care, patient safety, sickness absence and job dissatisfaction. Workload such as staffing levels were the most frequently examined factor in relation to burnout. High workload as well as time pressure is associated with emotional exhaustion.

Self-care and *The Code* (NMC, 2018b)

The previous section has introduced the concept and impact of stress through experiencing burnout. You would have recognised that this impacts not only on you as a healthcare practitioner, but impacts on the quality of care provided to patients and families. So how as a nursing associate can you look after yourself and why is it important?

The Code (2018b) specifically states your role in maintaining your health to undertake your role. You have a professional duty as well as an ethical obligation to adopt self-care as a duty to yourself in addition to a duty of care to your patients. A notable theory in examining the importance of self-care is Watson's theory of human caring. The core of the theory looks at humans who *cannot be separated from self, other, nature, and the larger workforce* (Watson, 1979). Self-care features heavily in that caring is an experience for both the patient and the nurse, as well as between all team members.

What does self-care mean to you?

Self-care is defined by the World Health Organization (2013) as the steps people take for themselves to establish and maintain their health. These steps are wide ranging from the lifestyle individuals lead to nutrition, impact of environmental factors and socio-economic factors that all impact on the ability to maintain health. While you may recognise the importance of self-care, implementation of self-care practices may sometimes prove more difficult in practice.

Nursing culture plays a prominent role in how as a nursing associate you may perceive the importance of looking after the self especially in the clinical environment. Permission from the self and others is usually a determining factor in how individuals perceive self-care and what steps they take to look after themselves. Recognition from managers, team members and the organisation towards prioritising self-care can enable healthcare workers to make it acceptable in everyday practice rather than to be implemented when individuals are stressed, experiencing burnout and fatigued.

Awareness around the 'self' is required to some extent to be able to recognise times when you may need to adopt the self-care measures. In nursing you may have heard of or applied in practice Maslow's Hierarchy of Needs (1943). Maslow conceptualised human needs as a pyramid with five levels in ascending order including the following:

1. Physiological needs
2. Safety
3. Belonging
4. Esteem
5. Self-actualisation

Maslow believed humans will work on meeting their unmet needs at a physiological level before attempting to meet the needs at the top of the pyramid which is self-actualisation. Self-actualisation refers to the human need of achieving their full potential including creative abilities and growth. For humans to meet their needs at the top of the pyramid they will work through each stage until their needs are met before they move to the next. So how does this apply to you as a nursing associate? Think about the Hierarchy of Needs in relation to your work and clinical practice. If your basic practice environment needs are not being met, you will be less likely to be motivated to progress to higher level functions. When referring to the work environment this includes your workload, scheduled breaks, staffing levels and overtime. As discussed earlier in the chapter, high workload, low staffing levels and a lack of breaks will result in job dissatisfaction, mental exhaustion and potentially burnout. As healthcare workers, when presented with low staffing levels, we may compensate by reluctantly taking regular breaks or not taking any at all. While this may seem like the 'safest' option this puts the safety of patients at risk. Lack of concentration results in impaired performance. In Maslow's Hierarchy of Needs, the need for air, food and water are essential for physiological functioning and taking regular breaks is an important element of meeting those basic needs in the work environment. As the stages of the pyramid progress through to esteem, belonging and self-actualisation, they mirror the core needs as identified in the Kings Fund (2021) *The Courage of Compassion* . As a nursing associate the need to feel part of a team (belonging) as well as having the autonomy to develop your professional practice through education and training are essential components of self-care.

For the following task you will have the opportunity to consider seven areas of self-care. This activity will allow you think about areas of your personal well-being that you may not have considered before.

Activity 7.2   Critical thinking

Review the seven areas of self-care listed below (Mental, Physical, Emotional, Spiritual, Social, Personal and Professional). Think about what each area means to you by providing a definition, then explore how you can maintain your self-care for that area. The first two areas have been completed for you, so you can think about the rest.

1. **Mental** – *Intellectually looking after your health can strengthen confidence in the workplace. Think about the following questions. What learning opportunities do you want to be part of? What can develop your confidence in your clinical practice? This can encourage belief in your own capabilities and know what they are.*

Activities might be:

- *attendance to training;*
- *participating in clinical supervision;*
- *mentoring students;*
- *reading journals;*
- *listening to podcasts on a topic of interest.*

2. **Physical** – *Exercise is a stress reducer as well as an energy booster. When you exercise, the body releases endorphins which are natural painkillers that can elevate mood and give you more confidence. Physical exercise can also promote good sleep.*

Activities you can do at work that can promote physical activity might be:

- *take a walk during your lunch break;*
- *using the stairs instead of the elevator;*
- *if you drive to work park your car further away from the car park;*
- *at home, taking a nap for 20 minutes can be extremely beneficial.*

Now add your own notes against the following five areas:

1. Emotional
2. Spiritual
3. Social
4. Personal
5. Professional

As this activity is based on your own critical thinking, no outline answer is provided at the end of this chapter.

Your well-being is in your control, while the above activity will make you think about self-care by adopting a holistic model of care. Having awareness of factors that may be influencing and preventing you from implementing self-care is self-awareness. Finding what works for you is important as implementing proactive approaches early in your career will allow you to build greater capacity to manage stress and increase resilience.

Emotional intelligence

Before discussing emotional intelligence (EI), it is worthwhile to define the term 'intelligence'. Traditionally you may associate intelligence with IQ performance; however, it has been recognised that IQ is only one of several types of intelligences. EI has its roots in social intelligence where human interactions and relationships are valued. Simply EI is described as having the ability to understand one's own emotions and others' feelings and emotions. This includes self-awareness as a core component of being able to impact relationships and how you manage this.

Ask yourself is empathy a required feature of working in healthcare? Many would agree without empathy, a therapeutic relationship cannot be developed, nor are you able to understand a situation from another person's perspective. Discussing the connection to EI do you think as a nursing associate you can have empathy without EI? Empathy can be defined as having the ability to understand and see someone else's viewpoint without judgement. You may ask how does this relate to your self-care? You can only implement approaches to self-care if you are able to identify when emotions are impacting behaviour and how this can positively or negatively impact others. As a registered nursing associate, you may lead a team of healthcare support workers, nursing associates in training and student nurses: your ability to connect with others easily in the workplace, read other people's feelings and responses accurately when interacting with them is a key feature of EI. These attributes have been deemed central to healthcare practice, in response influencing leadership abilities. It is understood the way in which emotions are experienced by individuals can affect the work of the team and performance. Emotions in this environment are not ignored but acknowledged and appreciated as there is an awareness of the importance of EI.

EI may be an asset to your path to self-care, as approaches such as reflective practice and self-evaluation will encourage you to explore your own experiences and practices by considering your emotions and behaviours.

Case study: Workload

Workload management is one of the causes of stress in the work environment. Imagine you are in the staff room at your workplace. This could be in any clinical setting – a hospital, community service, mental health unit, GP surgery, special school. You walk into the staffroom after being part of a conversation breaking bad news to a family of a palliative care patient. One of your colleagues is discussing her workload and she appears overwhelmed by a patient who is being rude to her, and the healthcare support staff. The patient keeps telling the nurse he wants a proper nurse to look after him. The nursing associate (NA) is tearful, but also states she is overwhelmed with her workload which is making her emotional. You are feeling equally as overwhelmed with the difficult conversation that you have been part of.

Research outside of nursing practice has demonstrated a correlation between emotional intelligence and important workplace outcomes such as job retention, stress management, burnout prevention and job satisfaction (Dal'Ora et al., 2020). More recently, the characteristics of EI have shown its central role within nursing. The above activity highlights the importance of having the ability of not only being aware of your own emotions and how it can impact others, but also the relevance of this in a profession where interpersonal skills are at the forefront of clinical delivery. An emotionally underdeveloped individual in the case study may possibly respond by not acknowledging the NA and her feelings about the rude patient and walk out of the room. Acknowledging the feelings and emotions of others through empathy and not allowing your own feelings to impact the interaction is what self-regulation is. This is where having a better understanding of your behavioural tendencies in situations of stress will allow you to work on your behavioural responses and adopt specific behaviours that will demonstrate you being emotionally aware. Team performance and morale is dependent on open and meaningful conversations between colleagues and especially for those in a leadership capacity. In your role as a nursing associate, the *Standards of Proficiency for Nursing Associates* (NMC, 2018a) state that to be an accountable professional you will be required to *recognise signs of vulnerability in themselves or their colleagues and the action required to minimise risks to health,* the achievement of this proficiency is closely related to proficiency 1.8, which asks you to explain the influence of EI and resilience on individuals. The above activity provides an insight into how being able to recognise the emotions of others and then using your own emotions to assist reasoning byhaving tough discussions can positively impact team dynamics, consequently reducing stress and burnout.

Approaches to develop EI

Developing EI in your practice is a skill that can be nurtured if you pay attention to yourself. This may not always be easy, however, now that you have been able to distinguish the components of EI, the following approaches will support you in developing EI in your practice.

Reflective practice

Reflective practice can enable healthcare practitioners to enhance their emotional intelligence skills, specifically self-awareness through insight. When reflecting on practice you will take a step back to make sense of what has happened and why. This process allows you to be more conscious of your emotions on yourself and others in situations. Being able to self-regulate your responses will allow adaptability in handling change.

Mindfulness

Mindfulness can be seen to recognise ourselves through thoughts, emotions and physical sensations through meditation. Gaining greater control over your thoughts to gain a perspective can consequently impact on relationships with patients and colleagues. Evidence suggests the use of mindfulness meditation can result in the reduction of stress and promotes self-care and self-compassion for healthcare professionals (Jiménez-Picón et al., 2021). While mindfulness practice has been seen to improve the well-being of the healthcare worker, its function does not stop there. Constant practice of meditation can improve cognitive function, learning and memory and helps in reducing blood pressure and stress hormones (Green and Kinchen, 2021). Working in healthcare, you cannot always predict when stressful events may occur, however, the practice of mindfulness can prepare individuals to regulate emotions when situations occur.

As a nursing associate there are many apps that can be accessed to practise mindfulness. Have a look at your own organisation's health and well-being support, where you may be able to find out how to practise mindfulness. There are also useful activities available on the RCN's website that show how mindfulness can be practised. This can be accessed via the following web page: www.rcn.org.uk/healthy-workplace/healthy-you/time-and-space

Self-assessment

Self-assessment allows an individual to think about certain emotional intelligence (EI) statements and how they apply to them. There are many EI scales that can be used but it is important to understand the two main types introduced by Petrides and Furnham (2000), which are:

- Trait EI – this is a self-report measure of behaviours in an emotion-relevant situation, for example, when an individual is confronted with stress or an upset friend. While using this type of measurement, participants need to be mindful as people are not always good judges of their emotion-related abilities.

- Ability EI – this is a test of maximal performance; responses are measured that are deemed to be correct or incorrect. Participants will solve emotion-related problems. Ability-based measures give a good indication of individuals' ability to understand emotions and how they work.

When you research to find self-assessment scales to measure EI, you will come across many scales. The main task of these scales will help you to pinpoint which elements of EI you've mastered and which you need to develop.

Impact of change on well-being

The Kubler-Ross change curve

Understanding how change can impact well-being can be useful when processing emotions and behaviours. During the COVID-19 pandemic, healthcare practitioners experienced uncertainty which greatly impacted on health and well-being. How individuals process their emotions and their ability to respond can be illustrated by the 'change curve' derived from the work of Kubler-Ross (1969). This model is usually used in developing leadership capacity but is also a useful tool to apply when faced with unpredictable changes and situations in the workplace setting. Some of these changes may include restricting of a service, getting a new manager, moving to a new building, or even introducing new equipment/tools to undertake your job. Whatever the cause of the change it will follow the following five stages:

- denial;
- anger;
- bargaining;
- depression;
- acceptance.

When applying the 'change curve' the first stage is usually the most disruptive to our emotions when we first experience change. Individuals will move through each stage experiencing different emotions which will have an impact on how they behave. This is where the skills developed through emotional intelligence will provide a foundation for how you respond to the situation. It is also important to remember, progressing through the change curve is personal to everyone regardless of how resilient you are; it will take time. However, if you are faced with a similar change and you recognise your emotions and the process, that same change will be easier to progress through.

The following activity will allow you to apply the above stages of the change curve model to changes within the workplace environment.

Activity 7.3   Critical thinking

A new electronic health assessment form has been introduced for all healthcare staff to record and review patient assessment at your workplace. Staff were informed about the change, but the current health assessment form that is being used is fit for purpose and there are questions around why the change was needed. Time is required to implement the new form as it will need to be completed electronically when assessing patients.

Follow the instructions below to complete the critical thinking activity.

- Provide a definition of each stage of the change curve model.
- Now for each stage write how you may feel during this stage and what could be provided by your manager to support you during this stage.

An outline answer is provided at the end of this chapter.

Feelings during the early stages can impact productivity as employee reluctance to engage in new systems. Showing empathy and allowing individuals space to talk will support moving through the stages. As a nursing associate you will also be in the position of introducing change to healthcare practice through your leadership skills.

Resilience

Resilience is defined by the capacity in which someone recovers from difficult and tough situations. Setbacks are part of life whether in your personal or professional life. Having the ability to be resilient in situations of stress and change has a positive impact on mental and physical well-being. In healthcare, the relationship between resilience and burnout have been evidenced (Arrongate et al., 2017). Overcoming adversity and adapting in the workplace requires a build-up of personal resilience. This doesn't mean individuals will not experience negative emotional responses such as fear, anger and sadness to change, but because they have made an effort to be resilient, they can move through the change easily, experiencing better mental health.

Arguably, people can be faced with similar situations but how they deal with those situations will differ because there are different types of resilience.

These are:

- natural resilience – this is the resilience you are born with and that comes naturally;
- adaptive resilience – this type of resilience occurs when you are forced to change and adapt due to challenging situations;
- restored resilience – this is where you learn techniques to build resilience. This type of resilience will allow you to deal with past situations and deal with future situations by utilising skills you have learnt.

Recognising that there are different types of resilience means personal resilience can be learnt. Try the activity below to explore this further.

Activity 7.4   Research

This activity has two parts:
1. Watch the following Ted Talk:

Ted Talk: The three secrets of resilient people
www.youtube.com/watch?v=NWH8N-BvhAw&t=50s

(Continued)

(Continued)

2.   What resilience strategies were identified in the Ted Talk and how can you adapt those strategies in the workplace to impact your well-being?

An outline answer is provided at the end of the chapter.

When going through change or grief we may need reminding of what is good in our lives and what our strengths are. We can concentrate on all the things we are not good at doing, but praising ourselves on all the things we can do is something we do not do often enough. If you were asked to write down seven of your strengths in one minute, would you be able to do that? Confidence in recognising strengths and areas of development is a key skill in self-awareness. Strengthening your support system and knowing when to ask for help plays a vital role in problem solving when faced with adverse situations. Problem solving with others will provide the opportunity to self-reflect on recognising and acknowledging the situation and can form part of your resilience strategy. You may want to ask yourself; how do you feel about asking for help? Can you identify individuals within your organisation who can be approached? If not, can you identify the barriers that prevent you from asking for support. What can you do to overcome these barriers? Some individuals may find being adaptable gives them the flexibility in how they examine a situation. Recovering from a situation if you recognise some situations can be beyond your control will give you the resilience to cope with change.

This chapter has explored many key concepts in giving you the insight into how stress and adverse situations can impact on health and well-being. By using the key concepts discussed throughout the chapter, you can complete the below task. Looking after yourself is essential in being able to maintain your health and well-being as well as adhering to your professional standards.

Activity 7.5   Reflection

Reflect on what you have read in the chapter and create your own self-care plan. This will be individual to you so really think about what matters to you and how the goals you create will benefit you.

As this activity is based on your own reflection, no outline answer is provided at the end of this chapter.

Chapter summary

This chapter brings *Team Working and Professional Practice for Nursing Associates* to a conclusion. This chapter brings the concepts of resilience and maintaining your identity in professional practice to focus. Self-care is not a new concept but the benefits of this within healthcare have shown to have wide-ranging benefits on organisations through to the quality of care provided to patients. We all experience stress as part of life, but the chapter allows you to explore and recognise when stress is having a negative impact on health and well-being. You will be able to identify factors that impact on stress and how you can manage these negative stressors through prioritising your self-care. The activities will enable you to critically think about identifying resilience factors and how these can then be used to develop a self-care plan. It is always a good idea to further explore concepts such as emotional intelligence and how these can be developed by accessing measurement scales available online. Working in healthcare will mean you will come across situations that will require you to be aware of your behaviours and feelings. It is not always easy to put aside some emotional responses but as a healthcare professional, you are bound by your professional standards. Your professional regulator (NMC) has been the underpinning driver in how you need to maintain your professional practice as a nursing associate working across all four fields of healthcare.

Activities: Brief outline answers

Activity 7.1 Critical thinking (page 101)

Individual factors:

- personal characteristics – personality, self-esteem, sense of identity;
- personal events – stressful life events such as marriage, divorce, illness, death of a loved one, family demands;
- professional demands of caring, professional experience.

Workplace factors:

- staffing levels;
- workload;
- organisational culture – not taking regular breaks;
- professional identity;
- lack of support from management;
- hours of work.

Physical health:

- cardiovascular symptoms;
- muscle tension;
- gastrointestinal symptoms;
- high blood pressure;
- exhaustion;
- aches and pains;
- psychological impact;
- inability to concentrate;
- fatigue;
- burnout;
- depression;
- unmotivated, overwhelmed, unfocused;
- easily distracted;
- memory lapses;
- anxiety.

Activity 7.3 Critical thinking (page 110)

- **Denial** – stage of shock and denial, individual may use defence mechanisms to challenge the change. While the introduction of the new health assessment form may have been planned and it was communicated to individuals, time is needed for staff to adjust. Clear communication is required by managers/those introducing the change to ensure individuals are not overwhelmed. Give clear direction where support and further information can be obtained.
- **Anger** – during this stage the reality of the change has begun to sink in. Feelings of anger and resistance are common. Threats will be identified in relation to the change and if not managed correctly, issues can spiral out of control. Careful management of the situation is required through planning and preparation. There needs to be understanding of the impact on staff and what the issues to change are. Those initiating the change need to listen; in the scenario of the introduction of the new electronic health assessment, it may cause anger as the element of time to implement the system will require commitment. Preparation is also key as information regarding why the change is happening needs to be clearly communicated.
- **Bargaining** – once the individual has passed the anger stage, they will attempt to explore the alternatives to find a compromise. If supported well, individuals will be able to explore what the change can mean. If support is not provided this can lead to the next stage of depression.
- **Depression** – in this stage an individual may lose all hope, and demotivation will develop. It can be difficult not to take responses personally during this stage, therefore emotional intelligence can be a useful skill in identifying how your behaviours can impact others. Those implementing the change need to recognise the change may be difficult for individuals as they may be on an emotional journey. An example of this can be the threat of t change. Implementation of the electronic form may mean some experienced staff may need to upskill themselves to undertake a task that they may have previously been experienced to do.
- **Acceptance** – individuals will come to terms with the change by accepting it. While for some it will continue to be uncomfortable, with time the change will be embraced. Celebrating success of the change is beneficial as it will make things easier if the change occurred again.

Activity 7.4 Research (page 111)

Watching the Ted Talk video, you would have identified the following three strategies:

- Acceptance and acknowledgment of the situation as part of life.
- Focus on the things you can change. To do this you need to identify what you can change rather than focusing on what cannot be changed. This process is referred to as 'selection attention' in the TED talk.
- Lastly, is your response and how you deal with a situation causing you harm or helping you? This is self-awareness through being emotionally intelligent.

Further reading

Green, A and Kinchen, EV (2021) The effects of mindfulness meditation on stress and burnout in nursing. *Journal of Holistic Nursing*, 39(4): 356–368

The journal article explores if mindfulness-based stress reduction programs potentially reduce stress and burnout in nursing. Peer-reviewed research related to the impact of mindfulness was reviewed.

Smart, A Creighton, L (2022) Professionalism in nursing 3: The value of self-care for students. *Nursing Times*, 118(6): 45–47.

This article provides proactive approaches that can be implemented to improve well-being by spotting and addressing the symptoms of stress.

The Kings Fund (2021) *The Courage of Compassion: Supporting Nurses and Midwives to Deliver High-Quality Care*. Available at: www.kingsfund.org.uk/publications/courage-compassion-supporting-nurses-midwives

The report sets out recommendations designed to meet three work core needs that need to be met to ensure well-being and motivation at work.

References

Advanced Life Support Group (ALSG) (2016) *Advanced Paediatric Life Support: A Practical Approach to Emergencies*. Oxford: John Wiley and Sons.

Aggar, C, Bloomfield, J, Thomas, T and Koo, F (2017) A time management intervention using simulation to improve nursing students' preparedness for medication administration in the clinical setting: A quasi-experimental study. *Collegian*, 25(1): 105–111.

Andrews, H, Tierney, S and Seers, K (2020) Needing Permission: The experience of self-care and self-compassion in nursing: A constructivist grounded theory study. *International Journal of Nursing Studies*. Available at: https://doi.org/10.1016/j.ijnurstu.2019.103436

Arrogante, O and Aparicio-Zaldivar E, (2017) Burnout and health among critical care professionals: the mediational role of resilience. *Intensive and Critical Care Nursing*, 42: 110–5.1. Available at: https://doi.org/10.1016/j.iccn.2017.04.010

Bach, S and Grant, A (2015) *Communication and Interpersonal Skills in Nursing*. 3rd edition. London: SAGE.

Bach, S and Ellis, P (2011) *Leadership, Management and Team Working in Nursing*. London: SAGE.

Baillie, L and Black, S (2014) *Professional Values in Nursing*. 1st edition. Abingdon: Taylor and Francis

Barr, J and Dowding, L (2019) *Leadership in Healthcare*. 4th edition. London: SAGE.

Beauchamp, T and Childress, J (2013) *Principles of Biomedical Ethics*. 7th edition. Oxford: Oxford University Press.

Behrend, B, Finch, D, Emerick, C and Scoble, K (2006) Articulating professional nursing practice behaviors. *Journal of Nursing Administration*, 16(2): 20–24.

Brewin, P (2012) Communication: A holistic approach, in *Children's Respiratory Nursing*. West Sussex, UK: John Wiley and Sons.

Campbell, U (2020) Interdisciplinary relationship dynamics. *American Journal of Health – System Pharmacy*, 77 (6).

Chaffer, D (2016) *Effective Leadership: A Cure for the NHS*. Abingdon: Taylor & Francis.

Children Act 1989, c.41. Available at: www.legislation.gov.uk/ukpga/1989/41/contents

Crane, A Geoffery. (2020) Chasing mercury: The emotional and social pillars of high-performing teams, in *The Practitioner's Handbook of Project Performance*. 1st edition. Abingdon: Routledge.

Cuncic, A (2019) *How to Practice Active Listening*. Available at: www.verywellmind.com/what-is-active-listening-3024343

Dall'Ora, C, Ball, J, Reinus, M and Griffiths, P (2020) Burnout in nursing: A theoretical review. *Human Resources for Health*, 41.

References

Day-Calder, M (2016) How to be a good role model. *Nursing Standard*. Available at: https://rcni.com/nursing-standard/careers/career-advice/how-be-good-role-model-65961

Equality Act 2010, c15. Available at: www.legislation.gov.uk/ukpga/2010/15/contents

Fahrenwald, NL, Bassett, SD, Tschetter, L, Carson, PP, White, L, and Winterboer, VJ (2005) Teaching core nursing values, *Journal of Professional Nursing* 21(1), pages 46–51.

Frances, R (2013) *Report of the Mid Staffordshire NHS Foundation Trust Public Inquiry*. Available at: https://assets.publishing.service.gov.uk/government/uploads/system/uploads/attachment_data/file/279124/0947.pdf

Gluyas, H (2015) Effective communication and teamwork promotes patient safety. *Nursing Standard*, 29(49).

Green, A and Kinchen, EV (2021) The effects of mindfulness meditation on stress and burnout in nursing. *Journal of Holistic Nursing*, (4): 356–368.

Griffith, R and Tengnah, C (2020) *Law and Professional Issues in Nursing*. 5th edition. London: SAGE.

Hargie, O and Dickson, D (2004) *Skilled Interpersonal Communication: Research, Theory and Practice*. 4th edition. Abingdon: Routledge.

Harris, M (2020) *Understanding Person-Centred Care for Nursing Associates*. London: SAGE.

Harris, M (2021) *Understanding Person-Centred Care for Nursing Associates*. London: SAGE.

Health Education England (2019) *Traverse: Evaluation of Introduction of Nursing Associates. Phase 2*. Available at: www.hee.nhs.uk/sites/default/files/documents/15.1%20-%20Trainee%20Nursing%20Associate%20Year%202%20Evaluation%20Report_1.pdf

Health Education England (2020) *Person-Centred Approaches: Empowering People in Their Lives and Communities to Enable an Upgrade in Prevention, Well-being, Health, Care and Support*. Available at: www.skillsforhealth.org.uk/images/pdf/Person-Centred-Approaches-Framework.pdf

Howatson-Jones, L, Standing, M and Roberts, S (2015) *Patient Assessment and Care in Planning*. 2nd edition. London: SAGE.

Human Rights Act 1998, c.4. Available at: www.legislation.gov.uk/ukpga/1998/42/contents

Humphrey, A (1970) *SWOT Framework*. Stanford Research Institute (SRI).

Institute of Apprenticeships (2021) *Knowledge, Skills and Behaviours for Nursing Associates*. Available at: www.instituteforapprenticeships.org/apprenticeship-standards/nursing-associate-nmc-2018/

Jiménez-Picón N, Romero-Martín M, Ponce-Blandón JA, Ramirez-Baena L, Palomo-Lara JC, and Gómez-Salgado J. (2021) The relationship between mindfulness and emotional intelligence as a protective factor for healthcare professionals: systematic review. *International Journal of Environmental Research and Public Health*, 2018(10): 5491. Doi:10.3390/ijerph18105491. PMID: 34065519; PMCID: PMC8161054.

Jung, CG (2014) *Psychological Types*. Volume Six. Hove: Routledge.

Lake, D, Baerg, K, and Paslawki, T (2015) *Teamwork, Leadership and Communication: Collaboration Basics for Health Professionals*. Edmonton, Alberta: Brush Education.

Maslow, AH (1943). A theory of human motivation, in *Psychological Review*, 50(4): 430–437.

McCormack, B and McCance, T (2017) *Person-Centred Practice in Nursing and Health Care Theory and Practice*. 2nd ed. Sussex: Wiley Blackwell.

Mental Capacity Act 2005, c.9. Available at: www.legislation.gov.uk/ukpga/2005/9/contents

Mental Health Act 1983, c.20. Available at: www.legislation.gov.uk/ukpga/1983/20/contents

Mulder, P (2018) *What Is Active Listening?* Available at: https://www.toolshero.com/communication-skills/active-listening/

National Voices (2017) *Person-Centred Care in 2017. Evidence from Service Users*. Available at: https://www.nationalvoices.org.uk/sites/default/files/public/publications/person-centred_care_in_2017_-_national_voices.pdf

NHS Digital (2022) *NHS Workforce Statistics – April 2022* (Including selected provisional statistics for May 2022). Available at: https://digital.nhs.uk/data-and-information/publications/statistical/nhs-workforce-statistics/april-2022

NHS England (2018) *Comprehensive Model of Personalised Care* . Available at: www.england.nhs.uk/personalisedcare/comprehensive-model-of-personalised-care/

Nursing and Midwifery Council (NMC) (2015) *The Professional Duty of Candour*. Available at: www.nmc.org.uk/standards/guidance/the-professional-duty-of-candour/read-the-professional-duty-of-candour/

Nursing and Midwifery Council (NMC) (2018a) *Standards of Proficiency for Nursing Associates*. Available at: www.nmc.org.uk/globalassets/sitedocuments/education-standards/nursing-associates-proficiency-standards.pdf

Nursing and Midwifery Council (NMC) (2018b) *The Code: Professional Standards of Practice and Behaviour for Nurses, Midwives and Nursing Associates*. Available at: www.nmc.org.uk/standards/code/

Nursing and Midwifery Council (NMC) (2019) *Blog: Role Differences Between Nursing Associates and Nurses*. Available at: https://www.nmc.org.uk/news/news-and-updates/blog-whats-a-nursing-associate/#:~:text=While%20nursing%20associates%20will%20contribute,within%20the%20integrated%20care%20team

Petrides, KV, & Furnham, A (2000). On the dimensional structure of emotional intelligence. *Personality and Individual Differences*, 29: 313–320. Available at: http://dx.doi.org/10.1016/S0191-8869(99)00195-6

Price, P (2019) *Delivering Person-Centred Care in Nursing*. London: SAGE.

Reeves, S, Lewin, S, Espin, S and Zwarenstein, M (2010) *Interprofessional Teamwork for Health and Social Care*. Oxford: John Wiley and Sons.

Robson, W (2017) Tools and techniques to improve teamwork and avoid patient harm. *Nursing Times*, 113(1), pages 24–27.

Rowe, G, Ellis, S, Gee, R, Graham, G, Henderson, M, Barnes, J, Counihan, C and Carter-Bennett, J (2020) *The Handbook for Nursing Associates and Assistant Practitioners*. 2nd edition. London: SAGE.

Senyuva, E, Kaya, H, Isik, B and Bodur, G (2013) Relationship between self-compassion and emotional intelligence in nursing students. *International Journal of Nursing Practice* 20 (6): 588–596.

Spurling, l (2004) *An Introduction to Psychodynamic Counselling.* New York, NY: Palgrave Macmillan.

Slusser, M, Garcia, LI, Reed, C and McGinnis, PQ (2018) *Foundations of Interprofessional Collaborative Practice in Healthcare.* London: Elsevier.

Sullivan, E and Decker, P (2005) *Effective Leadership and Management in Nursing.* 6th edition. Upper Saddle River, NJ: Prentice Hall.

Takase M, and Teraoka S, (2011) Development of the holistic nursing competence scale. *Nursing and Health Sciences,* 13: 396–403. DOI: 10.1111/j.1442-2018.2011.00631

Terry, L (2020) Understanding and applying different personality types in healthcare communication. *Nursing Standard,* 35 (7), pages 27–34.

The Kings Fund (2021) *The Courage of Compassion: Supporting Nurses and Midwives to Deliver High-Quality Care.* Available at www.kingsfund.org.uk/publications/courage-compassion-supporting-nurses-midwives

Tuckman, B (1965). Developmental sequence in small groups. *Psychological Bulletin,* 63(6): 384–399. Available at: doi:10.1037/h0022100

Vrbnjak, D, Denieffe, S, O'Gorman, C, and Pajnkihar, M (2016) Barriers to reporting medication errors and near misses among nurses: A systematic review. *International Journal of Nursing Studies,* Vol.63, pages 162–117.

Watson, J (1979). *Nursing: The Philosophy and Science of Caring.* Boston, MA: Little, Brown.

Williams, J, Perry, L and Watkins, C (2019) *Stroke Nursing.* 2nd ed. Oxford: John Wiley and Sons.

World Alliance for Patient Safety (2005). *WHO Draft Guidelines for Adverse Event Reporting and Learning Systems: From Information to Action.* Geneva: World Health Organization.

World Health Organization (WHO) (2013). *Self Care for Health. A Handbook for Community Workers and Volunteers.* Available at: http://apps.who.int/iris/bitstream/handle/10665/205887/B5084.pdf?sequence=1&isAllowed=y

Zeller, JM and Levin, PF (2013) Mindfulness interventions to reduce stress among nursing personnel: An occupational health perspective. *Workplace Health & Safety,* 61(2): pages 85–89. DOI: 10.1177/216507991306100207

Index

Locators in **bold** refer to tables.